BECOMING GOOD STEWARDS
OF ANTIBIOTICS

BECOMING GOOD STEWARDS of ANTIBIOTICS

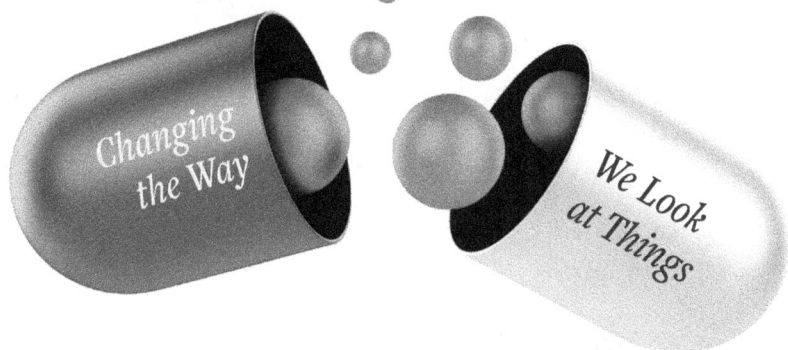

Changing the Way

We Look at Things

DR. PETER PATTERSON

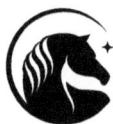

Cheval Press

BECOMING GOOD STEWARDS OF ANTIBIOTICS
Changing the Way We Look at Things
First Edition

ISBN   979-8-9890491-3-4   *Hardcover*
979-8-9890491-7-2   *Paperback*
979-8-9890491-8-9   *eBook*
979-8-9890491-9-6   *Audiobook*

LCCN   2024909951

*This book would never have been written
but for the stories told by the elderly to their
doctors, nurses, housekeepers, and me.*

*These true-life stories of the rampant—and
sometimes deadly—overuse of antibiotics are
shocking and, at the same time, inspiring.*

*This book is dedicated to all those who
told the truth about antibiotics.*

CONTENTS

FOREWORD

by Dr. Buffy Lloyd-Krejci

In 2016, I found myself at a state Healthcare-Associated Infections (HAI) conference, unaware of the profound revelation that awaited me. It was there, amidst a dynamic group of health care professionals, that I first encountered Dr. Patterson and his ominous discourse on the impending post-antibiotic era. His words struck a chord within me, unraveling a narrative transcending generations of medical practice.

Dr. Patterson, a third-generation physician, took the stage, his words resonating with urgency as he painted a stark picture of the looming post-antibiotic era. It was a term unfamiliar to many, myself included, yet its implications were staggering.

Dr. Patterson began with a poignant reflection on the transformative impact of penicillin, a beacon of hope in the fight against infections during his grandfather's era. But with this miracle drug came unforeseen consequences—overuse and the rapid emergence of antibiotic resistance. As he unveiled a timeline of antibiotic development juxtaposed with the rise of resistance, it became clear: we were witnessing a race against time, one in which humanity could ill afford to lose.

It was during this presentation that the seeds of change were sown within me. Dr. Patterson's decades of experience and the tangible success of his stewardship program spoke volumes. The revelation that facilities implementing his approach had eradicated *Clostridioides difficile* infections by simply curbing inappropriate antibiotic prescriptions was nothing short of astounding. Here was a beacon of hope amidst the escalating threat of multidrug-resistant organisms (MDROs).

As an epidemiologist specializing in long-term care, I had long grappled with the complexities of MDROs, particularly within nursing homes. Dr. Patterson's advocacy to address this challenge head-on struck a chord with me. His program wasn't just a suggestion; it was a clarion call for action—one that resonated not only with health care providers but also with families impacted by the repercussions of antibiotic misuse.

This book, a culmination of Dr. Patterson's expertise and insights, is a vital resource for all stakeholders in the health care landscape. Whether you're a nursing home operator, a prescriber, or a concerned family member, the principles outlined within these pages are indispensable. Transitioning from a culture of "just in case" prescribing to "just in time" interventions demands collective commitment and informed decision-making. Dr. Patterson's methodology, laced with practical examples and humor, guides facilities through an eight-step journey toward implementing effective antibiotic stewardship.

Central to Dr. Patterson's approach is the notion of leveraging common sense and diagnostics to guide antibiotic prescriptions judiciously. By empowering nurses with effective communication strategies and furnishing policymakers with actionable policies, he advocates for a paradigm shift in how we approach antibiotic use. The consequences of inaction are dire, as evidenced by the burgeoning threat of MDROs like *Candida auris*. With the Centers for Disease Control and Prevention (CDC) echoing Dr. Patterson's call to arms, the imperative for change has never been clearer.

We stand at a precipice, grappling with the specter of antibiotic resistance that looms ever larger on the horizon. The escalating measures to combat MDROs, from heightened infection control protocols to the uncomfortable reality of frequent culturing, underscore the urgency of our predicament. Dr. Patterson's impassioned plea serves as a rallying cry—a reminder that the time for complacency has long passed.

Antibiotic-resistant organisms encroach upon our communities, threatening lives and livelihoods with each passing day.

Yet, in the face of this formidable challenge, there remains hope. Through concerted efforts and unwavering resolve, we can stem the tide of antibiotic resistance. But the journey begins now, with each of us committing to become stewards of antibiotics—guardians of a precious resource upon which countless lives depend.

As you embark on this transformative journey through the pages of this book, I urge you to heed Dr. Patterson's wisdom. For the fate of antibiotics—and indeed, the future of health care itself—hangs in the balance. Together, let us rise to the occasion, for the stakes could not be higher.

Buffy Lloyd-Krejci, DrPH, CIC, LTC-CIP, is a leading authority on infection prevention in the long-term care industry. Her firm, IPCWell, delivers in-person gap analysis, training, and support to nursing homes across the country.

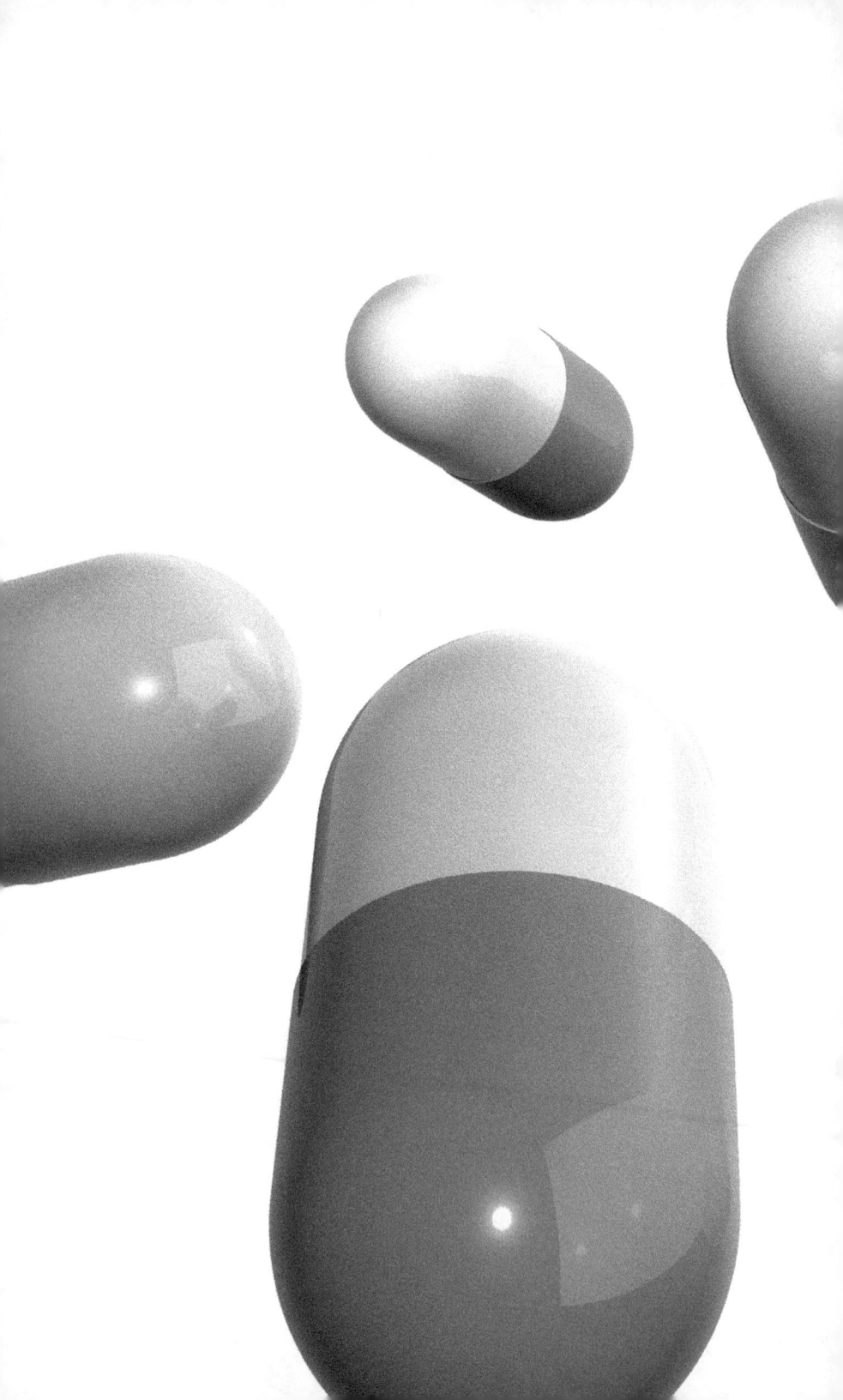

PART 1

THE
SEA OF
ANTIBIOTICS

We are awash in a sea of antibiotics. The words of my colleague, Stan Deresinski, MD FIDSA, head of the Stanford Antimicrobial Stewardship Program, echoed in my head as I sat listening to a panel of infectious disease experts. I was attending a seminar populated with the best and brightest in infectious disease control, listening to some very impressive speakers discuss the vaccines they'd been developing in an attempt to treat multidrug-resistant organisms (MDROs).

Along with describing their vaccines, these experts also called for more research to determine the cause of the antibiotic resistance that was, in their words, "suddenly" plaguing patients in long-term care facilities across the world. They went on about the issue at length, but the more they talked, the more I was struck by what they didn't say. They didn't say this resistance is a manifestation of what I call the post-antibiotic era. They didn't say that widespread antibiotic resistance is a full-fledged but little-talked-about public health emergency. They didn't say that vaccines are not the answer to this problem. And they certainly didn't say that more research is a waste of time and energy because we already know the root cause of all this resistance: the overuse of antibiotics.

It was disheartening, but not surprising. I've devoted the last thirty years of my professional life to addressing this problem, and what I've found, over and over, is that antibiotics are deeply ingrained in our culture. Furthermore, we all—health care professionals, administrators, patients, and family members alike—share the blame in their overuse. But we can't afford to be complacent in letting this problem continue. We *must* become good stewards and take action to both preserve and restore antibiotic effectiveness. The consequences if we don't are almost unthinkable.

Once we tip into the post-antibiotic era—when antibiotic resistance is the norm rather than the exception—things like open-heart surgery or major cancer surgeries [where antibiotics are so necessary to prevent infections before they have a chance to gain a foothold] will no longer be life-saving measures. Instead, they will become dangerous procedures. Fatality rates will skyrocket because, quite simply, antibiotics will no longer work. And nobody will be safe from this phenomenon: everyone, from children to senior citizens, has the potential to be affected.

Pulling back from the abyss won't be easy. It will require a complete paradigm shift—a sea change in the ideas and values we've all lived with for so long.

When my father graduated from medical school in 1942, we were at the dawn of the penicillin era, and it was a game-changer. To put its impact into perspective, because of penicillin, if you were wounded in the battle of Normandy, you had a 2 percent chance of dying of a wound infection. Compare that to the Civil War less than a hundred years earlier; if you were wounded in that war, you had a 30 percent chance of dying from an infection. No wonder antibiotics were hailed as miracle drugs!

They weren't just miracles for wounded troops, either. As antibiotics began to trickle out from the military to civilians, people with illnesses that were previously considered almost universally fatal—things like pneumonia, for example—could be cured. There didn't seem to be a downside to antibiotics, and pretty soon, doctors were prescribing them anytime they even *suspected* a patient had an infection. After all, what was the harm? Nobody knew then that antibiotic resistance would become such a huge problem; indeed, being a "good doctor" meant getting in front of any possible infection before it could take hold. Physicians were like gunslingers, and antibiotics were their weapon of choice.

Little has changed in the ensuing decades. In fact, most of us take this approach to the prescribing of antibiotics for granted, and very few people have spoken up against it.

One such person who did will remain forever branded in my memory. It was 1967. I was twenty-one years old, in medical school, taking a class from George Goldsand, MD, an expert in infectious diseases. Over forty years later, I still remember him saying, "The main problem in infectious disease today is people receiving antibiotics for infections *they do not have.*"

At the time, it didn't seem to apply to me. I was young, trying to finish my program so I could get out into the world and start helping people, and his words just didn't seem relevant. Plus, they flew in the face of conventional wisdom. But years later, when I started focusing on antibiotic resistance and stewardship, his words came flooding back: *The main problem in infectious disease today is people receiving antibiotics for infections they do not have.* Undoubtedly, that was true when I was twenty-one, and it's even more true today.

That's why I wrote this book. Far too many people— health care providers and patients alike—step over the truth of that statement like it's garbage in the street. They don't want to look at it, they don't want to acknowledge

THE SEA OF ANTIBIOTICS

it, and they certainly don't want to deal with it. And that's a problem, because it means the root cause of widespread antibiotic resistance isn't being addressed in a meaningful way. As a result, the issue just keeps getting worse and worse.

It's time for that stop.

Practitioners must learn to resist the urge to prescribe antibiotics "just in case." Those who work in long-term care must be willing to stop antibiotic use if a patient comes back from the hospital on an antibiotic for an infection they don't have. Nurses must learn to be more discerning about how they relay information to prescribers. Facilities must take steps to move the needle on antibiotic use. And patients and families must pledge to become antibiotic guardians.

None of this will be easy. However, it is all vitally necessary if we are to pull back from the brink of the disaster that's looming. Luckily, I've spent the past thirty years learning how to help everyone become better antibiotic stewards. No matter what role you play—patient, family member, nurse, facility administrator, or prescriber—this book will help guide you through how you can make a difference. And trust me, you *can* make a difference. Overuse of antibiotics is everyone's problem. It's not just about you, or your loved one, or your patient: antibiotic use in one person potentially affects *everyone* in their community.

It's time to wake up. Time to tell the truth and to accept the truth. Time to focus on antibiotic use by clinical syndrome. Time to concentrate on syndrome-focused data collection and reporting. And time to come up with alternatives to "just in case" antibiotic use. If we can do that— if we can bring the world to its senses and get people everywhere to stop overusing antibiotics—resistance *will* unwind. I've seen it over and over in facilities I've consulted for: they implement the strong stewardship program I describe in this book, and within a few months, antibiotic resistance begins to decline.

The time to avert the post-antibiotic-era disaster is running out, but if we take action now, we can prevent this tragedy from coming to pass. It starts with accepting the truth—that the vast majority of people receive antibiotics for infections they do not have—and then putting a truly strong, novel, and effective antibiotic stewardship program into place to prevent antibiotic overuse from driving us further into the post-antibiotic era.

While antibiotic resistance affects us all, it's beyond the scope of this book to talk about antibiotic overuse in every population. So I'll focus on my specialty: senior populations in long-term care facilities. But the underlying message is the same for everyone. Whether we are health care professionals or lay people, we must all be more intentional about antibiotic stewardship. That means, if you're a prescriber in a hospital or outpatient clinic, stop using antibiotics "just in case." If you're a nurse or a CNA, stop encouraging prescribers to give "just in case" antibiotics. And if you're a patient or the family member of a patient, stop with the "just in case" scenarios, too. In every instance, only prescribe or take antibiotics when they are truly warranted.

I know—this runs counter to everything we've been led to believe about how to use antibiotics. But as you'll see throughout the book, it's possible to adopt a mindset of antibiotic stewardship. And we must, for all our sakes.

Ready? Me too. Let's dive in.

1

ARE YOU SURE IT'S A UTI?

'LL NEVER FORGET THE MOMENT I HAD MY FIRST REAL wakeup call about the flagrant overuse of antibiotics. It was, of all days, April Fool's Day. I was working as lab director for a startup mobile diagnostics laboratory in Scottsdale, Arizona. Coming into that role, I certainly wasn't spreading the antibiotic stewardship gospel like I do now. But on that particular day, I was looking at our Laboratory Information System (LIS) to review the microbiology reports for people who had been receiving antibiotics for chronic urinary tract infections (UTIs). This was nothing new—I reviewed those reports regularly as part of my job. But on that particular day, I decided to look back at the progressive resistance over the past two years.

As I looked through the records, I noticed something shocking: the original urine cultures (those taken two years prior) showed S's (indicating sensitivity to antibiotics) for all antibiotics. There were no R's (which indicate resistance) to be seen. After a few months of receiving regular cycles of antibiotics, however, patients started exhibiting a few R's scattered amongst the S's. And within two years, many patients exhibited all R's, with only a few (or no) S's to be seen. In other words, after regular rounds of antibiotics to treat what were thought to be chronic UTIs, people had so much multidrug resistance that there were *no antibiotics left* that were capable of treating their infections. Those patients were effectively in their own post-antibiotic era.

It got worse. I soon realized these patients—some of whom were on regular doses of antibiotics for years—often didn't even meet the complete clinical case definition of a UTI. In other words, they were being treated, as Dr. Goldsand had said all those years ago, for infections *they did not have*, and the consequences of this were profound.

This indicated a sobering new reality, especially because there was a time when widespread antibiotic resistance wasn't an issue. When my father was practicing, for instance, in the

1950s and 1960s, new antibiotics were coming out almost every year. Those times are long gone. Now, the pipeline of new drugs has run dry, and any new antibiotics are really just massages of existing molecules. That's why we must all change the way we think. We have to set the bar higher for when we will and when we will not use antibiotics. Otherwise, just like the patients I was looking at that April Fool's Day, we will find ourselves universally in the post-antibiotic era...and the repercussions of that will be dire.

TURNING BACK THE TIDE

After my April Fool's wakeup call, something else happened that had a further impact on my commitment to antibiotic stewardship. I began working at Glencroft, a large long-term care campus in Arizona. My mission: to help them implement an effective stewardship program. Indeed, my time at Glencroft planted the seeds for the program I'm going to share with you in this book. It was in its nascent stages, though; I knew what we needed to do—stop giving antibiotics for infections people didn't have—but I wasn't sure exactly how to go about doing that. Luckily, I had someone who proved to be a valuable ally: a woman named Mary Matesan.

Mary was the assistant director of nursing (ADON) at Glencroft. No-nonsense and direct, she immediately understood the problem when I explained the patterns of increasing resistance I had seen. One day, she called me on the phone: "Dr. Pete, I don't know why we have all these urinary tract infections. Something's going on here."

I reviewed the data and then met with her. She was exactly right. Something was going on. The so-called urinary tract infections weren't infections at all. They didn't fulfill a complete case definition as defined by the McGeer Criteria for Urinary Tract Infection Surveillance.[1] To put it more succinctly, these weren't UTIs at all. Instead, they were the much more common asymptomatic bacteriuria (ASB).

Once Mary understood what was happening, she sprang into action. Anytime someone ordered a urine culture, she would confront them: "Why did you order that urine culture? Tell me exactly what was going on with that patient that caused you to make that decision." And let me tell you, the response, "Because that patient was confused," or "Their urine was dark/foul/stinky" wasn't good enough for her. Pretty soon, because of her efforts, the number of urine cultures began to go down. And not long after that, antibiotic resistance began to drop, as the following image illustrates:

[1] "Revised McGeer Criteria or Infection Surveillance Checklist," https://www.pharmacy.umaryland.edu/media/SOP/wwwpharmacyumarylandedu/centers/lamy/antimicrobial-stewardship/mcgeer-criteria-for-infection-surveillance-checklist_form.pdf, accessed March 2, 2024.

180-Bed SNF Stewardship Results 2015

Metric	4Q 2014	1Q 2015	2Q 2015	3Q 2015	4Q 2015	
Urine C&S orders	94	63	26	27	21	←
Urine C&S positive	65	46	12	16	10	
Days of UTI Antibiotic Therapy		268			85	
C. difficile orders	12	15	6	3	9	
C. difficile positive	7	4	4	0	0	←
ESBL + urine isolates	21	7	4	4	4	←

CASE DEFINITIONS MATTER

The situation at Glencroft wasn't unique—most cases of presumed UTI are actually ASB. By definition, ASB is when bacteria are present in the urine at levels often regarded as clinically significant (up to >100,000 colonies/ml) but, crucially, the patient exhibits *no or minimal symptoms related to the urinary tract.* As you now know, and as Mary found out that day, a significant proportion of antibiotic prescriptions for "UTIs" are driven by the misinterpretation of ASB as a treatable infection. It's not, and giving antibiotics to treat ASB does nothing except increase resistance to those drugs.

There are several common ways that ASB can masquerade as an infection. It may show up as a "positive" culture, which then leads to the diagnosis of UTI and a resulting antibiotic prescription. This is especially common in patients with altered mental status when they have a "positive" urinalysis/culture & sensitivity (UA/C&S). Or a "positive" UA/C&S may seem to predict the risk of invasive infection. While potentially concerning, none of these fit the case definition of a UTI:[2]

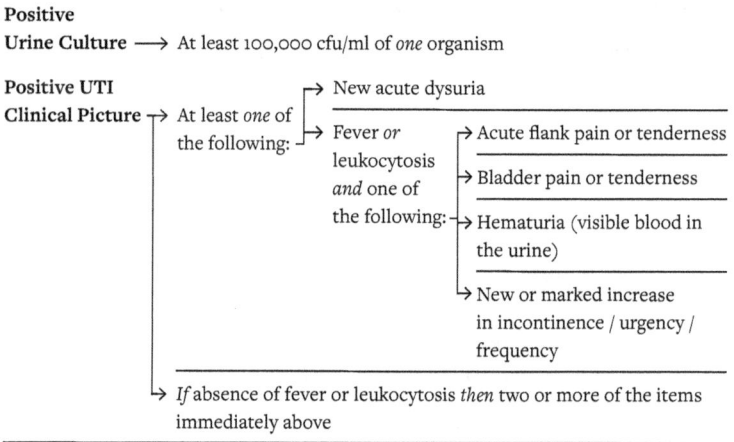

Positive
Urine Culture ⟶ At least 100,000 cfu/ml of *one* organism

Positive UTI
Clinical Picture ⟶ At least *one* of the following:
- → New acute dysuria
- → Fever *or* leukocytosis *and* one of the following:
  - → Acute flank pain or tenderness
  - → Bladder pain or tenderness
  - → Hematuria (visible blood in the urine)
  - → New or marked increase in incontinence / urgency / frequency
- → *If* absence of fever or leukocytosis *then* two or more of the items immediately above

ASB isn't the only time that antibiotics are given for a presumed UTI. If you're a prescriber, I bet the following scenario—I call it the "elevator ambush"—sounds familiar. You're heading to your rounds in the facility. As the elevator doors open and you prepare to step off, you're met with a cadre of

---

2 "Revised McGeer Criteria."

steely-eyed people: a nurse, maybe a CNA, and a family member or two of one of the residents. Their mission? Get an antibiotic for their patient or loved one's presumed UTI.

Sound familiar? Yep, I thought so. And how about this one? A family member corners you as you're walking down the corridor and says, "My mother isn't like other people. She knows when she has a UTI. She can just *tell*. And so, if my mother tells you that she has a UTI, just give her the antibiotic she always takes. Don't waste time with all those tests!" And of course, this applies to family members who say the same thing about their fathers, brothers, sisters, aunts, or uncles.

Look, I get it. In instances like these, the easiest thing to do is often to give the antibiotic. However, easier isn't always better. Rather than writing a prescription, take time to educate the family members and the nurses about the difference between ASB and UTI. Let them know the impact that occurs when antibiotics are given for infections that people don't have. And then, tell them that you have a better approach: the UTI protocol.

THE UTI PROTOCOL

The UTI protocol is simple: push fluids and take vitals twice per day for forty-eight hours. At the end of those forty-eight hours, reassess the resident to determine if they fit the case definition for UTI. If they do, then give them antibiotics. If they don't (as is the case the vast majority of the time), then don't. How easy is that? You're "treating" the symptoms while avoiding inappropriate antibiotic use. And what you're most likely to find, in the words of one of my friends and colleagues, is that "at the end of forty-eight hours, there's nothing left to treat!"

The UTI protocol avoids any risk that antibiotics will be given empirically. In essence, empirical antibiotics are those that are prescribed when you don't know the name of the organism or its susceptibilities. This should be avoided in low-likelihood scenarios. Take the time to see if the body can handle whatever's happening on its own. If it can't, make sure you know exactly what you're dealing with and what's indicated to treat it. That's being a good steward of antibiotics; after all, stewardship doesn't mean *never* using antibiotics, it means only using them when they are actually indicated.

When it comes to antibiotics and UTIs, one way your facility can help your residents' loved ones get on board with the antibiotic stewardship program is through education. I regularly provide a short article I wrote called "Are You Sure Your Loved One Has a UTI?" to facilities I consult for so they can hand it out to family members and visitors. Feel free to use this in your own facility; just remember to put it on your own letterhead. Here is the full text for your reference:

. . . .

Are You Sure Your Loved One Has a UTI?
How Taking Antibiotics When They Are Not
Needed Can Cause More Harm Than Good

At <Facility Name>, our goal is to provide the best care possible. We believe in working together with our residents and families so you feel we are meeting the needs of your loved one. In this spirit we are writing to share new findings about antibiotic resistance and urinary tract infection (UTI).

Today there is national and worldwide attention focused on antibiotic resistance and its root cause—unnecessary use of antibiotics. One of the most frequent reasons seniors are given antibiotics are UTIs. Yet studies are showing that many of these UTIs are misdiagnosed—a result of confusion between normal resident bacteria and those causing infection.

It turns out there are many bacteria living in and on our bodies that cause no harm. In fact, these bacteria—which outnumber our human cells 10-to-1—are needed for us to live, digest our food, and have our immune systems function properly. Some of these bacteria live naturally in the bladder without causing any pain or symptoms. This is called asymptomatic bacteriuria, which can be present in half or more of seniors living in long-term care settings.

In the past when a urine specimen tested positive for bacteria—even when no symptoms were present—doctors were taught to treat this bacteriuria with antibiotics, just in case they might eliminate the cause of any future problems. We now know this is unnecessary and often harmful.

Multiple studies have shown that giving antibiotics in this situation does not help. It does not prevent UTIs or urinary sepsis. It does not improve bladder control. It does not help memory problems or balance. In fact, the main result of treating asymptomatic patients with antibiotics is complications. Antibiotics here can kill "friendly" bacteria leading to vaginal yeast overgrowth or severe diarrhea from overgrowth of toxic bacteria in the bowel. Yet the most sinister unseen complication is the emergence of resistant bacteria. Their resistance is the result of repeated cycles of antibiotic treatment. These resistant bacteria have come to predominate in our world—now a global public health emergency more important than AIDS or Ebola virus.

As a family member, you are an important care partner for your loved one. By understanding the risks of using antibiotics when not needed you help us to provide good, safe care. Antibiotics should be used only when the doctor or nurse practitioner is sure that there is an infection. We no longer use antibiotics "just in case." When antibiotics are prescribed or not prescribed, we want you to feel comfortable asking questions.

The safest care happens when the entire team understands and follows the most current recommendations. If you would like more information please ask one of our nurses for the <Facility Name> packet on antibiotics and UTI.

. . . .

GET STAFF BUY-IN

Of course, residents' loved ones aren't the only people who need to be on board for your antibiotic stewardship program to work. Your entire staff, from prescribers to nurses, CNAs, and even housekeepers need to buy in, too, which means they need to be educated both about the problem (that the majority of people are given antibiotics they don't need) and what to do about it.

This is especially important when it comes to nurses. That's because nurses drive 75 percent of antibiotic use by both what they say to prescribers (i.e., MDs and NPs) and how they say it. So get your nursing staff together and walk them through the truth about antibiotics and resistance. Then guide them in understanding how they can impact antibiotic usage by going through a series of mock conversations with them about the right way and the wrong way to talk to prescribers about a resident's presumed UTI.

Let me explain. The wrong (but all too common) way for nurses to discuss a resident's symptoms with a prescriber goes something like this: "This is Nurse Smith from <facility name> calling. We have a culture here on Mrs. Jones that was done on the weekend, and it's growing E. coli at 100,000 colonies. What do you want to use?"

Most of the time when I engage in these mock conversations with nurses, they chuckle when I share the "wrong-way" scenario with them. They know it's the most common way to approach prescribers, and they can readily understand why it almost universally results in antibiotics being ordered, whether or not they're really needed.

Once they're done laughing, we talk about the *right* way to talk to a prescriber. That goes something like this: "Hello, doc. So with regard to Mrs. Jones, she's fine. I just did her vitals, and she's well. She's not running a temperature, and she has no symptoms. For some reason, I think she was a little confused on the weekend, so they ordered a culture. It's back with E. coli with over 100,000 colonies, pan sensitive. I don't think this is a urinary tract infection, but I wanted to let you know and give you a chance to go on our *suspect-UTI* protocol, where we push fluids and do vitals twice a day for forty-eight hours and then reassess." That conversation, as you can imagine, results in a very different outcome than the first one.

Teaching your nurses the right way to talk to prescribers is a great start when it comes to antibiotic stewardship. Don't stop there, though: empower your nurses to push back against inappropriate antibiotic use if necessary. How? By training them to pull out the big guns.

Let's say a doctor has prescribed antibiotics for what is most likely ASB. The nurse needs to look that doctor in the eye and say to them, "Now, about your patient, Mrs. Jones, who is on Rocephin for a urinary tract infection...we are required by federal regulation to report about the use of antibiotics. I want you to know that this case does not meet the definition of infection."

If that feels too harsh, walk them through how to soften it: "Gee, doctor, we're now required by these darn federal regulations to do this reporting. It's not my fault, but I have to do it!" Either way, the point is made, and the prescriber knows that they better sit up and take notice.

EDUCATE YOUR PRESCRIBERS

It's important to spend some time educating your prescribers, too. Just like with the nurses, start by telling them the truth about antibiotics and resistance. Acknowledge that they were probably trained to believe that the mark of a good clinician lies in how fast they can sniff out the early signs of an infection and get the patient on a powerful antibiotic. Then let them know there is new evidence that demonstrates that many of the things that were previously thought to be infections actually aren't (hello, ASB!). Bottom line, disrupt their built-in urge to give an antibiotic when they're unsure as to whether it's needed. Remind them that the only time an antibiotic should be given is when a patient meets the case definition for an infection, and that giving antibiotics empirically is no longer a best practice.

Even your CNAs and housekeepers need to get involved, which is a lesson that was driven home to me one day when a facility called me after receiving an immediate jeopardy (IJ) from a Centers for Medicare and Medicaid Services (CMS) surveyor. Part of the way to resolve the matter was to fix their antibiotic stewardship program. So they brought me in. I'll never forget it: there was a set of bleachers where their staff were all sitting. It reminded me of a high school basketball game. Every single seat was taken. The medical director was there, the nurses, and about midway up were all the CNAs and housekeepers.

I started out the way I always do, telling the audience the truth about antibiotics and resistance and explaining why this issue is so important. The CNAs and housekeepers were rapt. And you know what? It soon became apparent from their questions and comments that they were one of the keys to getting the families on board. They are in the residents' rooms every single day. They chat with them and their visitors, and are often the first to notice when something might be wrong. They're also the first line of defense against the elevator ambush. They can talk to families who are concerned about whether their loved one has a UTI, and they can give them some insight into the dangers of giving antibiotics unnecessarily. In other words, if you want to reduce inappropriate antibiotic use in your facility, you're going to need the support of these critical staff members.

ANTIBIOTIC STEWARDSHIP AND THE SEPSIS PROTOCOL

Before we wrap up our discussion about presumed UTIs and antibiotics, there's one more scenario we have to discuss: Residents visiting an emergency room and getting antibiotics for—you guessed it—an infection they don't have (and, often, for something unrelated to the original complaint). This happens all the time, but why? And more importantly, what can you do to prevent it? To answer those questions, let's take a trip into the mind of an ER doc.

Doctors in the emergency room are marching to the beat of a loud, powerful—and perhaps surprising—drum: preventing sepsis. The END SEPSIS and STOP SEPSIS campaigns introduced various measures, including World Sepsis Day[3] and "Rory's Regulations," to address unidentified and untreated sepsis in hospitals.[4] As a result of these initiatives, sepsis protocols[5] were put in place to guide physicians to utilize early delivery of antibiotics for any individual that may have an infection. In most instances, this "early delivery" means getting antibiotics into patients within sixty minutes of being admitted to the emergency room. And *that* means— say it with me now!—patients in the ER frequently receive antibiotics for infections they may not have.

A CASE STUDY: MRS. CLARK

You can imagine how that plays out for residents in long-term care facilities. But just to make sure we're all on the same page and to show you how far this can go, let me share a real-life case study of one such resident. We'll call her Mrs. Clark.

Mrs. Clark was in her 70s. Diagnosed with primary progressive aphasia (PPA) and dementia, she was a memory care resident at a facility in North Carolina. PPA damages parts of the brain that control speech and language; by the time Mrs.

---

3   "World Sepsis Day: stop sepsis, save lives!" https://www.esicm.org/world-sepsis-day-stop-sepsis-save-lives/, accessed February 16, 2024.

4   "National Sepsis Policy," END SEPSIS: The Legacy of Rory Staunton, https://www.endsepsis.org/national-sepsis-policy/, accessed December 8th, 2023.

5   "Sepsis Protocols," END SEPSIS: The Legacy of Rory Staunton, https://www.endsepsis.org/work/sepsis-protocols/, accessed December 8th, 2023.

Clark arrived at the facility, it had robbed her of the ability to say all but a few words. In fact, the only things she said were "Amazon," "lizard," and her name. Despite her lack of speech, she was able to inflect her voice to convey her mood, and the staff had gotten to know her well. They knew when she was happy, and they knew when she was sad. They also knew when she was more confused than normal.

On one such occasion, only a few months after first coming to the facility, a CNA noticed that Mrs. Clark seemed "confused and out of sorts." She was sent to the ER, where a UA&C was performed. The urinalysis showed a positive nitrite and a positive leukocyte esterase. That's it. It didn't match the case definition for UTI, but the ER put her on an antibiotic anyway. (Hear that drumbeat? Gotta stop any chance of sepsis—and knock out any potential UTI, too!)

Ten hours later, she was back at the facility. Three days later, she was back to normal. "Must have been the antibiotic," the CNAs and nurses thought. "Thank goodness we caught that infection in time!"

About six weeks later, Mrs. Clark's urine was dark and foul. This time, the facility's health care personnel did a UA&C, and shocker of shockers: tens of thousands of colonies of bacteria grew! Back onto antibiotics she went. Once again, a few days passed, and her urine returned to normal. Another "crisis" averted.

But then, two months later, the same thing happened: dark urine, colonies of bacteria, and an antibiotic prescription. And then again three months later, after staff determined that Mrs. Clark was acting confused. Every few months, the cycle repeated: Mrs. Clark's confusion or "foul" urine triggered a urinalysis and/or a trip to the ER, and the result of those events was, invariably, more antibiotics. Importantly, though, Mrs. Clark *never met the case definition for UTI.*

Over the course of the next eighteen months, Mrs. Clark was put on antibiotics no less than *nine times* for infections she did not have. Her medical records were eye-opening: drugs like TMP/SMX (trimethoprim/sulfamethoxazole), Nitrofurantoin, Cefdinir, Ciprofloxacin, and Levofloxacin regularly appeared. She generally improved after being placed on the antibiotics, but that was simply an artifact of timing: she would have improved anyway. And lest you think that maybe the antibiotics *were* necessary, remember: at no point during the year did she ever meet the case definition for UTI. She was sent to the hospital because she was confused (ironic, because she had dementia), or dark urine, or some bacteria. That's it. And her story is far from unique. Residents across the country—and indeed, the world—are being given antibiotics for infections they do not have, and every time they are, it drives us one step closer to the post-antibiotic era.

I often joke that one of my fantasies in life is to meet a gaggle of emergency room physicians walking down the street. I'd throw myself down in front of them and make them trip over me. As they picked themselves up and dusted themselves off, I'd sit up, look them dead in the eye, and say, "Now that I have your attention, can we talk?"

The group of us would grab a delicious lunch (in my fantasy, I'd trip them right outside of my favorite restaurant) and have a conversation about ASB and how it isn't urosepsis based on the urinalysis. And then—because hey, this is my fantasy, so I get to imagine it however I want—they'd nod with understanding and find a better way to deal with sepsis than prescribing "just in case" antibiotics.

Look, all jokes aside, I understand that sepsis is serious. But so is widespread antibiotic resistance. I don't have all the answers about how to balance the need to avoid sepsis against the need to avoid inappropriate antibiotic use, but I do know how to start: before sending a resident to the ER because they're confused or their urine is foul or smelly, use the UTI protocol. If things don't improve after forty-eight hours, or if the resident's symptoms end up meeting the case definition, then by all means: send them to the hospital or start them on an antibiotic. But don't come in guns blazing. When it comes to antibiotics, shooting first and asking questions later is *not* the way to go.

So there you have it: my thoughts—based on decades of experience—about how to reduce the chances that ASB masquerading as UTI will lead to inappropriate antibiotic use. Implementing the strategies laid out in this chapter will go a long way toward bolstering your antibiotic stewardship program. But an effective program also focuses on collecting the correct data—the key word being *correct*.

Look, it doesn't do any good to collect information about how many tons of penicillin you used last quarter. Instead, you need to track diagnostic test results (EMR): how many new antibiotics were started, how many new diagnostic tests were performed, and how many people were put on isolation. Then capture comparison data: how many people were treated (i.e. given an antibiotic) versus the number of people who actually met the case definition. Finally, create performance metrics to track over time. If you do all of this, not only will you be adhering to the letter of the law that says you must have an antibiotic stewardship program in place, but you'll be adhering to the spirit of the law as well—you'll have a stewardship program in place that's actually moving the needle forward in reducing the antibiotic prescribing that leads to widespread antibiotic resistance.

Along with presumed UTIs, presumed pneumonia and presumed pressure wound infections are the most common reasons for inappropriate antibiotic use in long-term care facilities. We'll get into each of those in more detail in the next chapter, and then we'll go over how to set up a strong antibiotic stewardship program at your own long-term care facility (including ways to address MDROs among your residents). Finally, we'll look at some real-life case studies so you can see what to do and what mistakes to avoid.

KEY TAKEAWAYS

- The main problem in infectious disease today is people receiving antibiotics for infections they do not have.
- The vast majority of presumed urinary tract infections are actually asymptomatic bacteriuria.
- Before prescribing antibiotics for a urinary tract infection, make sure it meets the case definition for a UTI.
- Getting your facility's prescribers, nurses, CNAs, and housekeepers to buy into your antibiotic stewardship program will greatly increase its effectiveness.
- Educating your residents' family members about antibiotic stewardship reduces the likelihood that they'll demand antibiotics for infections their loved ones don't actually have.

- Before sending a patient to the ER, consider running the UTI protocol to see if they improve without antibiotic usage.
- Along with education, make sure your antibiotic stewardship program is set up to collect and report the proper data.

2

PRESUMED PNEUMONIA *and* PRESUMED PRESSURE WOUND INFECTIONS

N THE LAST CHAPTER, WE FOCUSED ON ONE OF THE biggest culprits for the overuse of antibiotics in long-term care facilities: asymptomatic bacteriuria (ASB) masquerading as a urinary tract infection (UTI). Determine when to test for UTI; get clear on what actions to take while you're waiting for results; decide when antibiotics are indicated and when they are not; and teach your staff how to talk to prescribers, residents, and families about ASB, UTI, and antibiotics...and you'll significantly curb the overuse of antibiotics at your facility. I know, because I've seen it happen firsthand, time and time again. And I can tell you unequivocally: The trickle effect of this kind of change is profound. In a nutshell, when you get your arms around the UTI issue, antibiotic resistance goes down for both individual residents and the facility community as a whole.

Obviously, though, UTIs are only a part of the problem—a significant part, yes, but still only part. To avoid careening headfirst into the post-antibiotic era, we have to wrap our arms around the *whole* issue. So let's turn our attention to another piece of the pie: prescribing antibiotics for what can only be called *presumed* pneumonia. Why presumed? Because, like UTIs, many people are diagnosed with what is "presumed" to be pneumonia even when what they have doesn't meet the case definition.

YOU CAN'T FIND PNEUMONIA ON AN X-RAY

Let me tell you a story that illustrates this phenomenon perfectly. I had been called in to help a facility improve their antibiotic stewardship program. I'd just finished telling some of the staff the truth about antibiotics, and we were taking a short break. I was standing over by the coffee machine, getting ready to pour myself a cup, when a nurse came up to me. "You know," she said with a big grin, "I was thinking about what you said about people getting prescribed antibiotics for infections they don't have. It reminded me: recently, I overheard one of our residents saying to a family member, 'I woke up with a little cough the other day, so they sent me in for a chest X-ray. I had no idea I had pneumonia until they came and told me they found it on the X-ray!'"

I laughed when the nurse told me that. "Now, you gotta level with me," I said to her. "When you see a real pneumonia patient, do they ever say things like that?"

"No!" she said. "When people have pneumonia, they are damn sick with it! There's no way they have it and don't realize they're ill."

It was a funny story—the best one I've ever heard about presumed pneumonia. But it was far from unique. Just like ASB and UTI, people get diagnosed with pneumonia all the time, even though what they have doesn't meet the case definition. It happens so frequently that it's a universal joke: a bad one, to be sure, but still very real. And you know why? Because so many of the people who are diagnosed with pneumonia *don't have it*. At least, not according to the case definition.

Let's play a little game. In your next meeting with your facility's medical personnel, I want to invite you to ask the room a simple question: In their experience, how many people who actually have pneumonia say, "I hardly knew I was sick!"?

You already know the answer, don't you? *Nobody* says that. Zero. Zilch. Zippola. When someone *really* has pneumonia, they have a cough that often produces yellowish, greenish, or bloody mucus. They generally have fever and chills. They may experience shortness of breath or rapid, shallow breathing. They also have chest pain, low energy, loss of appetite, and fatigue. And in older people especially, they might experience confusion. In other words, it's obvious that they're sick. Like, really sick. But that's an example of how deep in our culture antibiotics go. As soon as something funny shows up on an X-ray, many doctors and nurse practitioners react by prescribing an antibiotic *just in case*...and each time they do, antibiotic resistance goes up.

I understand why it happens. Remember, antibiotics are entrenched in our collective subconscious as miracle drugs. So when a radiologist sees a new infiltrate, or a prescriber notices that a sputum culture is growing all sorts of little bugs, their immediate response is to hit that patient with an antibiotic.

We have to do better.

CHANGE THE WAY YOU LOOK AT THINGS

I was recently at a conference where one of the speakers said something that completely changed my entire way of thinking about antibiotics. After thirty years, that doesn't happen very often, so when it does, I sit up and take notice. I'll never forget her words: *When you change the way you look at things, the things you look at change.* The truth of what she said slapped me right across the face. She was right!

So often before changing how they do things, the medical community demands to see evidence that supports making the change. That's backwards. Take ending the "just in case" use of antibiotics, for example. Demanding to see the evidence first is the wrong way to go. First, you need to recognize the uncomfortable truth: Our actions are driving us ever closer to the post-antibiotic era and all the dangers that go along with it. When we let that truth sink into our hearts, minds, and souls, *how* we look at things changes. All of a sudden, we see antibiotic overuse everywhere.

When that happens, *what* we look at starts to change. Suddenly, we're no longer focused on getting someone onto antibiotics just in case they have an infection. No, we're looking for evidence that people truly have infections in the first place. Then and *only then* do we act to give them antibiotics.

It was a brilliant insight—one that I want you to keep in mind throughout the rest of the book. For now, though, let's return to our discussion of pneumonia. More specifically, let's examine the case definition of pneumonia and what it means for residents of long-term care facilities.

PNEUMONIA CASE DEFINITION

To meet the case definition for pneumonia,[6] a person must have:

- A positive chest x-ray
- Leukocytosis *or* fever *and* one of the following:
  - New or increased cough
  - New or increased purulent sputum
  - Hypoxemia (sat. <94 percent on air or >3 percent on oxygen)
  - Respiratory rate >25/min
  - New or changed lung exam findings
  - Pleuritic chest pain
- In the absence of leukocytosis or fever, two or more of the items listed above must be present.

This case definition makes it quite clear that you cannot appropriately diagnose pneumonia from a chest X-ray and dry cough alone. Nor can you rely solely on a sputum culture. These cultures are notoriously unreliable: below the level of the trachea, the respiratory tract is essentially bacteria-free. However, when someone coughs up mucus for the culture, it

---

6   "Revised McGeer Criteria."

goes through the oropharynx, which is chock-full of organisms. It's essentially a sewer; there's nothing sterile about it! And so, of course, all sorts of lovely little microorganisms will start growing on the culture plate.

I can't emphasize this enough: A sputum culture in isolation is not good enough to diagnose pneumonia. As for chest X-rays? After decades in this field, I can tell you beyond a shadow of a doubt that elderly people have pretty junky chests. There's bound to be *something* going on in there. Too often, though, when a resident has a dry cough, their prescriber simply orders an X-ray. When they do, the radiologist might note a new infiltrate and say, "This could be atelectasis, congestive heart failure, or pneumonia." As soon as the p-word shows up, the nurse will call the doctor and say, "The X-ray report says it could be pneumonia"...and all hell breaks loose.

By now, you know exactly what's going to happen. The prescriber thinks, "I better put them on antibiotics just in case." Then they tell the nurse to put the patient on ciprofloxacin or to give them a gram of Rocephin. It hurts like hell when you give it intramuscularly, but they aren't worried about that. They're worried about nipping pneumonia in the bud just in case their patient has it.

REPLACE "JUST IN CASE" WITH "JUST IN TIME"

You know what? We need to replace "just in case" with "just in time." In other words, we need to change the way we look at things so that the things we look at change.

Imagine this scenario—aspirational, perhaps, but it's within reach with the right mindset: A patient has a dry, unproductive cough and complains of minor chest pain. The chest X-ray reveals a new infiltrate. However, the patient doesn't exhibit any other major symptoms and doesn't meet the case definition. So the prescriber elects to wait and monitor the situation for a period of twenty-four or forty-eight hours. The patient's pain, not to mention their cough, recedes without antibiotics.

I'm telling you right now, that dream can become reality. How? Only reach for antibiotics when someone has been properly diagnosed according to the case definition. Until it has been absolutely proven that they have pneumonia, assume they don't. If they do meet the case definition, give antibiotics in time to stop the infection. Otherwise, conduct the tests necessary to determine what you're actually dealing with, then treat accordingly.

To make this aspirational story the norm and not just a pipe dream, everyone at your facility needs to get on board with your stewardship program when it comes to commonly misdiagnosed issues like presumed pneumonia. Take your nursing staff, for example. Just like with UTIs, there is a better way for nurses to talk with prescribers when pneumonia is suspected. For example, rather than simply stating the radiology report said the X-ray could be indicative of pneumonia, the nurse could say something like, "You know that chest X-ray you ordered the other day because Mrs. J had a dry cough? It's come back, and the radiologist did note that it contained a new infiltrate that might indicate pneumonia. However, I've been monitoring her and her temperature has been normal. She doesn't have a productive cough, and it doesn't look like the case definition for pneumonia has been met. It looks like it's just an unresolved infiltrate. I'll continue to monitor her."

By approaching it this way, the nurse demonstrates that he or she is on top of the situation. As a result, the prescriber feels comfortable that, at least for the moment, no prescription is needed. And most importantly, the patient isn't given antibiotics unnecessarily. Win-win-win!

PRESSURE WOUND INFECTIONS

Along with presumed UTIs and presumed pneumonia, there is one more issue that contributes significantly to the overprescribing of antibiotics in long-term care facilities: presumed pressure wound infections. Many times, prescribers will use antibiotics in patients with pressure wounds because they are concerned the infection will get down into the bone and cause osteomyelitis. However, with a pressure wound infection, there's no valid culture you can do to determine if an infection is present.

Let's say that someone is riding a motorcycle. Unfortunately, on this particular day, they aren't wearing their good leather pants. They take a corner too fast and tumble, badly scraping the side of their leg and tearing the skin off. Any culture that's taken from the wound will grow all manner of lovely things. And why wouldn't it? Microorganisms love that kind of environment. Unfortunately, though, that means the culture report has no relationship to an actual infection. Yes, it's a positive culture, but it doesn't fulfill the case definition for a pressure wound infection.

Of course, we're primarily talking about long-term care facilities, so chances are our residents aren't speeding around on motorcycles. So let's consider another, more common scenario: pressure ulcers.

Pressure wounds (or pressure ulcers, as they're sometimes called) are far more likely to occur when people are immobile, incontinent, have lost physical feeling, have blood flow problems, and/or have thin or weakened skin. These risk factors make long-term care facility residents some of the most at-risk for pressure wounds. Because they are so prevalent among this population, pressure wounds round out our list of the "big three" culprits that often lead to inappropriate antibiotic use in nursing homes.

Why? Well, if a resident has a pressure ulcer, the fear sometimes is that it will lead to an infection that will spread throughout the body and eventually lead to death. As you can imagine, if the prescriber is worried about that, they may prescribe antibiotics to stop the spread of infection before it even begins—another "just in case" tactic that often does more harm than good.

CASE DEFINITION FOR PRESSURE WOUND INFECTIONS

Just like with UTI and pneumonia, there is another way. And just like with the first two, it starts with properly identifying whether a pressure sore requires antibiotics in the first place. Granted, this can be a bit trickier to assess than UTI or pneumonia, but the case definition is still clear. Let's break it down.

The clinical picture of positive wound infection[7] requires either of the following:

---

7   Modified from "Revised McGeer Criteria."

- A stage 3 or 4 pressure wound assessment
- Leukocytosis *or* fever *and* at least three of the following:
  - Redness at site
  - Heat at site
  - Swelling at site
  - Pain at site
  - Tenderness at site
  - Serous drainage at site
- In the absence of leukocytosis or fever, then at least four of the above must be present. Also, note that positive wound purulence requires pus to be present at the site *and* a positive culture.

Along with this case definition, prescribers should bear the four stages of pressure wounds in mind.[8]

- **Stage I**: The mildest stage. In stage I, the pressure wound only affects the upper layer of the skin. The most common symptoms at this stage include pain, burning, and/or itching. The pressure wound area may also feel different from the skin around it (i.e., warmer, cooler, firmer, or softer).

---

8   Deanna Altomara, "Pressure Sores: Treatment, Stages, and Symptoms," WebMD, https://www.webmd.com/skin-problems-and-treatments/pressure-sores-4-stages.

- **Stage II:** At this stage, the pressure wound starts to dig below the skin's surface. The symptoms of this stage include swelling, warmth, pain, and (in some instances) clear fluid or pus oozing from the wound. The skin is broken or may look like a pus-filled blister.

- **Stage III:** In the third stage, the pressure ulcer has penetrated through the second layer of skin into the fat tissue. This is the first stage where the pressure wound begins to show clear signs of infection. It often has a bad odor, with red edges to the wound. Sometimes, the tissue in or surrounding the pressure wound is black, which is an indicator that the tissue has died.

- **Stage IV:** In the final (and most serious) stage, the pressure wound may have penetrated so deep that it affects muscles, ligaments, and bones. At this point, the skin has turned black and signs of infection—including red edges, pus, heat, odor, and/or drainage—are present. Bone, muscles, and tendons may also be visible.

Prescribing antibiotics to treat pressure wounds that are not infected falls under inappropriate antibiotic use. For example, in the first stage, antibiotics are not needed. Instead, the best way to address the pressure wound is to eliminate pressure in the affected area, wash the pressure wound with mild soap and water, and dry it gently. Let me say it again for the people in the back: At this point, because infection is not present, antibiotics shouldn't be, either.

As the stages progress, it doesn't automatically mean that antibiotics should be prescribed. Sometimes cleaning the wound, keeping it covered, and/or debriding it may be enough to address the problem. Of course, because infections and/or sepsis *can* occur, the pressure wound should be closely monitored, but using antibiotics "just in case" is not a good solution. Instead—just like anything else—use them "just in time."

To determine whether a pressure wound is infected, prescribers should use the case definition and the four stages I laid out above. They can also use a wound biopsy in conjunction with these criteria to diagnose wounds (especially those that are not responding to treatment).[9] Or, if a prescriber thinks they're dealing with osteomyelitis, they can do an imaging study that will show early destruction of the bone's surface.

No matter what they decide, the takeaway is the same: As with UTIs and pneumonia, prescribing antibiotics for a pressure wound "just in case"—especially when someone is in stage 1 or stage 2—is a bad idea.

---

9 *Physiopedia*, "Assessment of Wound Infection," accessed December 11, 2023, https://www.physio-pedia.com/Assessment_of_Wound_Infection.

GET THE NURSE AND PRESCRIBER INVOLVED

When determining the best course of action to address pressure wounds, the optimal approach is to get both a wound nurse *and* a wound doctor involved. Make sure they both understand there isn't a valid culture you can do to determine if there's an infection because the wound itself is a cesspool of microorganisms. Once they acknowledge that, there's a much greater chance that they'll avoid inappropriately prescribing and administering antibiotics.

I admit that many wound care prescribers don't immediately jump to systemic antibiotics. If they *do* use antibiotics, it's generally in gauze that contains Vaseline along with the antibiotic. They put it on the wound and then, when it's done its work, they pull it off and the wound is nice and clean, with no pus or debris. Yes, antibiotics were used, but they weren't systemic. Plus, they were used "just in time," not "just in case." That's the goal.

Let that sink in for a moment. Now, let's go back to the statement that made such an impact on me. *When you change the way you look at things, the things you look at change.* Whether you're dealing with UTI, pneumonia, or pressure wound infections, you need to change how you look at things. We all do. That's the key to changing the decisions we make—and when we do that, the positive results will start to pile up.

It all starts with shifting our mindset. That's the foundation for becoming a good antibiotic steward—and it's imperative if you want to successfully implement the antibiotic stewardship protocol I'm going to share with you starting in the next chapter.

KEY TAKEAWAYS

- Just like with UTIs, make sure people meet the case definition for pneumonia before prescribing antibiotics.
- Relying on chest x-rays to diagnose pneumonia often leads to inaccurate results.
- If a resident who has been prescribed antibiotics for pneumonia says they had "no idea" they were sick, chances are those antibiotics were prescribed inappropriately.
- Unlike UTIs and pneumonia, pressure wound infections are a little trickier to diagnose. Utilizing biopsies and the pressure wound assessment tool will help.
- Culturing wound tissue can lead prescribers to misdiagnose infection.
- To truly create a culture of antibiotic stewardship in your facility, remember: When you change the way you look at things, the things you look at change.

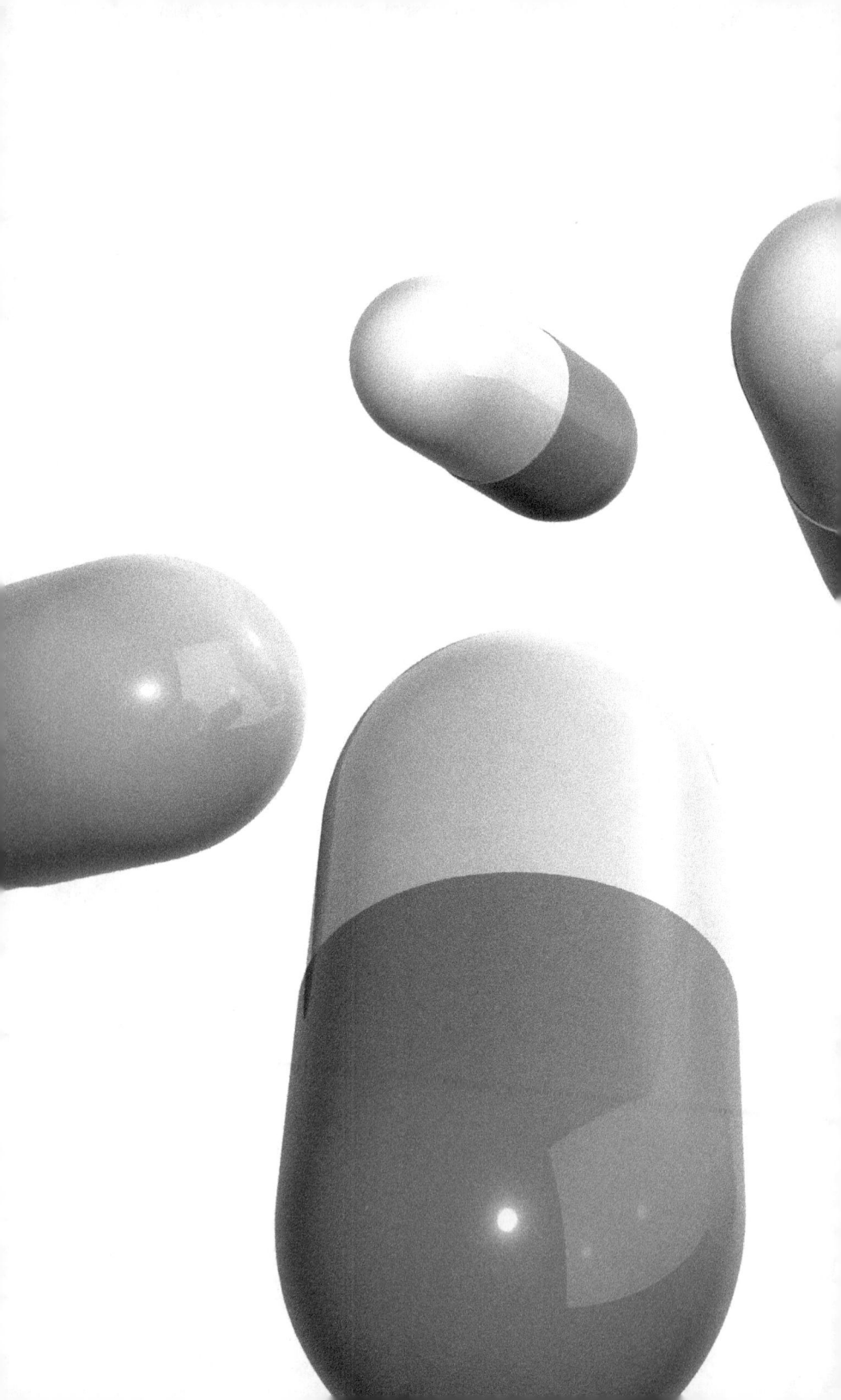

PART 2

IMPLEMENTING THE ANTIBIOTIC STEWARDSHIP PROTOCOL

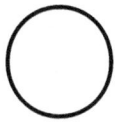

Over the last few chapters, we've seen how important it is for long-term care facilities to get a handle on antibiotic usage. However, a strong antibiotic stewardship program isn't just a way to prevent us sliding headfirst into the post-antibiotic era. It's also required under federal law. In 2015, the Centers for Disease Control and Prevention (CDC) published recommendations for nursing homes to establish antibiotic stewardship programs around seven core elements: leadership, accountability, drug expertise, action, tracking, reporting, and education (we'll talk more about how to meet these elements in chapter 4).[10]

Two years later, at the end of 2017, Centers for Medicare and Medicaid Services (CMS) began requiring participating nursing homes to have an antibiotic stewardship program "that includes antibiotic use protocols and a system to monitor antibiotic use."[11]

---

10 Caroline J. Fu et al., "Characteristics of Nursing Homes with Comprehensive Antibiotic Stewardship Programs, Results of a National Survey," *American Journal of Infection Control* 48, no. 1 (January 2020): 13–18, https://www.ncbi.nlm.nih.gov/pmc/articles/PMC6935405/.

11 Fu et al., "Characteristics of Nursing Homes."

Given that these regulations have been in place for years now, the likelihood that your facility has an antibiotic stewardship program is high. Whether or not it's effective is another story.

Look, I'm certainly not trying to take the wind out of your sails. However, in my years of experience, I've found that nursing homes struggle to create strong antibiotic stewardship programs more often than not. Despite having the best of intentions, there are so many other things to take care of—especially in our post-COVID world—that it's easy for a stewardship program to fall by the wayside.

If your facility is simply going through the motions of antibiotic stewardship, it's time to make a change. It's time for a *revival*. And the protocol I'm going to share with you is exactly that—a way to revive your stewardship program so that it's truly effective. And if you're starting from scratch, you're still in luck because the protocol works equally well for brand-new programs.

I've spent years developing and perfecting this protocol in real-world situations. Over time, I've come to realize that in order to be successful, you need to implement this protocol in a particular sequence of eight steps. I'll walk you through each of them in detail, but in a nutshell, here they are:

- **Step 1**: Cultivate interest
- **Step 2**: Conduct the senior team meeting
- **Step 3**: Send an announcement letter co-signed by the administrator, the director of nursing (DON), and the infection preventionist (IP)
- **Step 4**: Conduct training for prescribers, nurses, CNAs, and families
- **Step 5**: Conduct IP training
- **Step 6**: Send monthly/quarterly reports to the Quality Assurance Assessment (QAA) team
- **Step 7**: Communicate quarterly findings and next quarter's goals
- **Step 8**: Follow up daily/weekly with prescribers, nurses, and CNAs

Implementing these eight steps will significantly move the needle in terms of getting a handle on antibiotic usage in your facility—specifically, by reducing the number of inappropriate cultures and the use of inappropriate antibiotics. Why? Because, taken in their totality, the steps in the protocol focus on six main outcomes: telling the truth about antibiotics, focusing on antibiotic use by clinical syndrome, ensuring syndrome-focused data collection and reporting, capturing comparison data, offering alternatives to "just in case" antibiotic use, and providing in-service education.

When those outcomes are achieved, amazing things happen. We are able to *measure* antibiotic prescribing by syndrome. We are able to make antibiotic overuse *visible*. We are able to *minimize* overdiagnosis and over-treatment of presumed UTI, presumed pneumonia, and presumed pressure wound infections. Finally, we are able to *enhance* decision-making by prescribers, nurses, residents, and families in order to steer a transition in mindset.

Sounds good, right? I thought so. Let's dig in.

3

GETTING EVERYONE ON BOARD

BEFORE YOU CAN IMPLEMENT AN EFFECTIVE ANTI-biotic stewardship program, you need to get buy-in from everyone in your facility. And to do *that*, you need to cultivate interest in the program. That's what the first two steps in the implementation sequence—scheduling and holding the senior team meeting—are intended to do.

The senior team meeting is exactly what it sounds like: a meeting with the "senior triad" (administrator, medical director, and DON) at your facility. If possible, it's really help-ful to have a few other people there, too—specifically, the IP, Q/A nurse, and pharmacy consultant.

IT'S ALL ABOUT THE DATA

I suggest opening the meeting by telling the truth about anti-biotics, the same way I did for you at the start of this book. You can also remind the senior team that an antibiotic stew-ardship program is required under federal law. Then tell them that to successfully move the needle on antibiotic use, it's imperative to measure the *right* data.

At this point, it's a good idea to pause and make sure every-one is with you. Are they leaning forward and engaged? Do they look confused? Are their arms crossed while they stare daggers at you? Take a moment to gauge the various reactions of everyone in the room. If they're all with you, you can move forward. If not, spend some time identifying and discussing their concerns. Remember, the name of the game is cultivat-ing interest; fostering that right from the start is key to mak-ing the stewardship program effective.

When everyone is on the same page, go back to talking about the importance of collecting data and measuring out-comes. This is crucial: If you don't measure, you'll struggle to determine whether things are getting better, staying the same, or getting worse. And if you can't determine that, your program will fail. Remember, though, this step is all about cultivating interest and getting buy-in, so engaging in dialogue is important. Ask them some questions, including "What does our current program measure?" and "How do we measure it?"

Many times when you ask this, people will start talking about measuring how many pounds of particular antibiotics they used over the past quarter. Here's the thing, though: *That doesn't compel the right action*—and you can gently explain that to them. Then let them know what data *should* be collected:

- What was being treated each time an antibiotic was used
- Was it a genuine infection or an instance of a "presumed" diagnosis
- What percentage of diagnoses were for actual infections
- How many people received antibiotics for infections they didn't actually have
- How many days someone was given antibiotic therapy (both for true infections and for "just-in-case" scenarios)

To help the senior team wrap their heads around the importance of collecting the right data, it's helpful to talk about the three main culprits: presumed UTI, presumed pneumonia, and presumed pressure wound infections. Before you close

BECOMING GOOD STEWARDS OF ANTIBIOTICS

the meeting, make sure they understand how critical it is to verify that a patient meets the case definition for a given infection before antibiotics are prescribed.

THE ANNOUNCEMENT LETTER

Once the senior team is on board, you need to get the rest of the facility personnel to buy into your revival. To do that, you can utilize a powerful tool: the announcement letter.

The announcement letter is primarily intended to let everyone on staff know that the winds of change are blowing. It highlights that your facility's stewardship program is going through a revival; you aren't going to do things the same way anymore. No longer will "just-in-case" antibiotics be the law of the land. Instead, your facility is going to start measuring, collecting, and reporting relevant data about antibiotic usage. On top of that, distinguishing between cases that do and don't meet case definitions will be a priority, and every quarter, the findings will be reported to the senior team.

The entire senior team should sign the letter and disseminate it as widely as possible throughout the facility. This is key—it gives the letter teeth and demonstrates to people that this change is for real. It also gives facility staff the backing they need to stand by the new policies in the face of any resistance they may encounter.

For your convenience, here's a sample template of the announcement letter you can use as a model for your own letter (names are made up for the purposes of this example):

Dear [FACILITY NAME] prescriber,

As long-term care providers, we aspire to give our residents the highest quality care. To accomplish this goal, our community depends on us to provide care while adhering to recommended standards of evidence-based practice.

The COVID-19 pandemic disrupted our antibiotic stewardship program. A substantial increase in antibiotic prescribing became part of the pandemic. The [FACILITY NAME] leadership team is now implementing a post-COVID revival of antibiotic stewardship. There is renewed CMS attention to the requirement that facilities like ours regularly review antibiotic utilization and have protocols in place to promote optimal prescribing practices.

Under the revival protocol, the Stewardship Team will be gathering prescribing data from the EMR [NAME OF EMR]. Beginning immediately, antibiotic prescribing practices will be audited and reported quarterly to prescribers, the QA committee, and administration. The focus will be prescribing for presumed UTI, pneumonia, and pressure wound infections. We anticipate provision of these data each quarter will prove valuable to prescribers as an objective professional benchmark.

Thank you for your support of this post-COVID revival.

_____

John Andonov D.O., Medical Director

_____

Jackie Gallegos, Director of Nursing

_____

Heather Spiegel, Administrator

_____

Melissa Otero, Infection Preventionist

Once you've sent the letter out (and posted it throughout the facility for good measure), it's time to move on to the next step of implementation: training. There are four groups of people that need training and education: residents and their families, CNAs, nurses, and prescribers. Because each of these groups have different roles, responsibilities, needs, and goals, the training for each varies slightly. So let's break down the training for each of them, starting with residents and their families.

EDUCATING RESIDENTS AND FAMILIES

The best way to educate residents and their families is to talk to them about the importance of becoming good antibiotic stewards. Remember in chapter 1 when I shared the short article, "Are You Sure Your Loved One Has a UTI?" Distribute that to them, and include a letter explaining that your facility is committed to a strong antibiotic stewardship program that will keep them (or their loved one, if they're a family member) safe while at the same time reducing the inappropriate use of antibiotics. You can also include some information about the dangers of what will happen if we enter the post-antibiotic era. Finally, invite them to take the pledge to become good stewards of antibiotics (see the following page).

WHEN ARE ANTIBIOTICS APPROPRIATE?

You've undoubtedly heard this before, but given the propensity we all have to reach for antibiotics anytime we feel even just a little under the weather, I think it's worth taking just a moment to talk about when antibiotics are appropriate and when they're not. I'm going to give it to you straight: Antibiotics *only* work for certain bacterial infections, such as strep throat, some types of pneumonia, whooping cough, or

Becoming Good Stewards of Antibiotics

"We are awash in a sea of antibiotics."
—Dr. Stan Deresinski, Stanford Antibiotic Stewardship Program

The **root cause** of widespread antibiotic resistance:

- Overuse of antibiotics
- People receiving antibiotics for infections they do *not* actually have.

The **remedy**: Becoming good stewards of antibiotics:

- *Preserving* antibiotic effectiveness
- *Restoring* antibiotic effectiveness

The **culprits** in antibiotic overuse—*all* of us.

- Antibiotics (miracle drugs) are deeply embedded in our culture.

When You Change the Way You Look at Things, the Things You Look at Change.

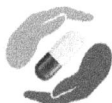

BECOME AN ANTIBIOTIC GUARDIAN

Keep Antibiotics Working

PLEDGE

"For infections that my body is good at fighting off on its own—like coughs, colds, sore throats, and flu—I pledge to treat the symptoms for five days rather than going to the doctor."

urinary tract infections (real ones, not ASB masquerading as UTI). They *do not work* for viral infections—think colds, gastroenteritis, sore throats (with the exception of strep), the flu, and most instances of bronchitis. Full stop. End of story. They are also not appropriate for some of the more common bacterial infections, such as sinus infections (caused by bacteria) and some ear infections. (And yes, I know many doctors prescribe antibiotics for sinus infections. In many instances, though, sinus infections aren't caused by bacteria; in those instances, antibiotics are inappropriate. Yet another reason prescribers should be crystal-clear about what they're treating before they start passing out prescriptions!) Giving antibiotics "just in case" for infections like these doesn't do any good, but it does cause harm.

We can all make a significant impact on antibiotic overuse by understanding and adhering to this. So the next time you, a patient, a resident, or a loved one has an infection, check to determine what kind of infection it is before you bring antibiotics into play. If it's something that antibiotics won't work for, treat it symptomatically, and let it run its course.

EDUCATING NURSES AND CNAS

Educating your staff about the antibiotic stewardship program requires a slightly different approach. Let's start with some ways to train nurses—who drive a significant portion of antibiotic use in facilities—and nursing assistants.

First, set up a mandatory in-service meeting with all of your nurses and CNAs (you may need to schedule several to make sure everyone has a chance to attend). Start the meeting by telling them the truth about antibiotics: the biggest problem in infectious disease today is people receiving antibiotics for infections they do not have. Then give them some examples. One of the best (and one that I frequently mention because it's so relatable) is to tell them the story of the overzealous family member that I shared in the first chapter: "*My* mother isn't like other people. *She* knows when she's getting a UTI. She can just *tell*. And so, if my mother tells you she has a UTI, just give her the antibiotic she always takes. Don't waste time on tests!"

Every nurse and CNA who has been working at a facility for any length of time can relate to this scenario. As they're nodding, tell them you understand that the natural inclination in a situation like this is to simply press the prescriber for an antibiotic to make the resident and family member happy. Now, though, things are going to be different. Remind them of the announcement letter, and tell them they have the senior team's support to approach the matter differently.

They can gently explain to the concerned family member that the facility's policy is to only prescribe antibiotics if someone meets the case definition for an infection. They can also remind them of the dangers of prescribing antibiotics for a nonexistent infection. Then they can reassure the family member that they are monitoring the resident and will take appropriate action based on what they find.

It's also helpful to give them a short course in microbiology. Talk about how many organisms we have in our body that are actually "friendly," despite what many people believe. A great example is E. coli. Most people think of E. coli as bad—and it can be, if it's out of balance in the body. But as the CDC clearly indicates: "E. coli bacteria normally live in the intestines of people and animals. Most E. coli are harmless and actually are an important part of a healthy human intestinal tract."[12] (Plus, E. coli makes steak taste good...and I'm all for that!) And E. coli is far from the only beneficial bacteria we have in the body; we have trillions of bacteria[13] that help us break down our food, regulate our moods, and perform a myriad of other functions.[14] Reminding your staff of

12 "E. coli: Questions & Answers," https://www.cdc.gov/ecoli/general/index.html, accessed February 16, 2024.

13 Ron Sender, Shai Fuchs, and Ron Milo, "Revised Estimates for the Number of Human and Bacteria Cells in the Body," PLOS Biology 14, no. 8 (August 2016): e1002533. https://www.ncbi.nlm.nih.gov/pmc/articles/PMC4991899/.

14 "Your Microbes and You: The Good, Bad and Ugly," NIH News in Health, November 2012, https://newsinhealth.nih.gov/2012/11/your-microbes-you, accessed February 16, 2024.

this—and of how the indiscriminate and inappropriate use of antibiotics affects bacteria and our microbiome—is a helpful exercise when it comes to changing your facility's culture around antibiotic use.

Once you've shared the truth with your nurses and CNAs and gone over some microbiology basics, take some time to discuss the strict case definitions for the "big three" (UTI, pneumonia, and pressure wound infections). When you do, make sure to share the McGeer criteria for each that I outlined earlier in the book.

After you've done all that, it's time to give them the tools they need to better communicate with the prescribers. Take a few minutes to role-play the "wrong way" and the "right way" to talk to doctors and nurse practitioners about the residents. I shared a few examples of these conversations in the first two chapters, but to refresh your memory, let's pretend that a nurse is talking to a prescriber about a resident with dark, foul urine.

First, the wrong way: "This is Nurse Jones calling you from <facility name>. We have a culture here on Mrs. Gilbert that was done on the weekend, and it's growing *E. coli* at 100,000 colonies. What do you want to use?"

Now, the right way: "Hi, doc. This is Nurse Jones from <facility name>. With regard to Mrs. Gilbert, she's fine. I just did her vitals, and she's well. She's not running a temperature, and she has no symptoms. For some reason, I think she had some foul urine on the weekend, so they ordered a culture. It's back with *E. coli* with over 100,000 colonies, pan sensitive. I don't think this is a urinary tract infection, but I wanted to let you know and give you a chance to go on our *suspect-UTI* protocol, where we push fluids and do vitals twice a day for forty-eight hours and then reassess."

Presented side-by-side, it should be readily apparent to both your nurses and your CNAs that the second approach results in a very different—and much better—outcome than the first.

Finally, use the in-service training to teach your nurses specifically about how to push back against inappropriate antibiotic use if they feel a prescriber isn't adhering to the policies of the stewardship program. Again, role-playing is a great way to do this. So let's pretend that a doctor or nurse practitioner prescribed antibiotics for a resident with a dry cough and an unidentified infiltrate. The nurse can call the prescriber and say something like, "I see that you want to put Mrs. Gilbert on an antibiotic for her cough and chest X-ray. She doesn't meet the case definition for pneumonia, and we're now required by federal regulations to report when people are put on antibiotics for suspect infections. It's not my fault, but I have to do it!" This is a great way to put the prescriber on notice without creating an unpleasant backlash for the nurse.

The in-service training is also a great time to go over how important it is to follow the UTI protocol and to share some information with your nurses and CNAs about asymptomatic bacteriuria and the many ways it can masquerade as UTI. As you do, remind them that the point of all this information is to support a culture shift within the entire facility from prescribing antibiotics "just in case" to prescribing them "just in time."

For your convenience, here's a helpful graphic outlining the training program that all of your staff should go through during the in-service:

Stewardship Protocol: Training Program
Targets: Prescribers, Nurses, All Staff

- The root cause of antibiotic resistance
- Clinically relevant microbiology—short course
- Standard definitions of UTI, PNA, pressure wounds: McGeer criteria applications
- Talking to prescribers—the effective way
- 48-hour observation pathway
- Asymptomatic bacteriuria (ASB) guidance
- Stewardship protocol in action
- Antibiotic Rx is in transition: *from* "just in case" *to* "just in time"

EDUCATING PRESCRIBERS

When it comes to educating prescribers, it's often difficult to get them all on-site at the same time for an in-service.

So it's best practice to put together a short handbook that explains the revised stewardship program and its principles. The handbook should include the signed announcement letter and clearly explain the truth about antibiotics. It should also tell the prescribers that your facility will be collecting, measuring, and reporting data about the use of antibiotics. To maximize its impact, the handbook should ideally be coauthored with the medical director. If the medical director doesn't have time to coauthor the handbook, get them to write a page or so describing the initial goals of the program (for example, eliminating empiric antibiotic use), then insert that page into the handbook so your prescribers see it. This step can serve to supplement and support the announcement letter and keep your antibiotic stewardship program top of mind.

Additionally, make sure the handbook clearly states that, despite their trained inclination to give an antibiotic "just in case," you expect them to only prescribe antibiotics to residents for infections they actually have. That means residents must meet the case definition for a given infection before antibiotics are used.

In the handbook, it may also be helpful to share the truism, "When you change the way you look at things, the things you look at change," along with a brief explanation of how they can look at antibiotics differently and what effect doing

BECOMING GOOD STEWARDS OF ANTIBIOTICS

so will have on the things they should be looking at. Finally, make sure the handbook clearly spells out the fact that, from here on out, one of the things you'll be looking at is how many antibiotics are given inappropriately. In other words, using antibiotics empirically will no longer be acceptable.

Once you've cultivated interest and gotten everyone on board, it's time to begin what is arguably the most important part of your antibiotic stewardship program: collecting, measuring, and reporting the data. So that's where we'll go next. See you in the next chapter!

KEY TAKEAWAYS

- Successfully implementing an antibiotic stewardship program requires buy-in from everyone at your facility, from the senior triad through to residents and their families.
- Creating an announcement letter and disseminating it widely is a great way to make sure your staff are on board with the stewardship program.
- Educating residents and their families about the importance of becoming good antibiotic stewards will make your program far more effective.
- Train your nurses and CNAs about the right way to discuss potential antibiotic use with prescribers.

- Creating a handbook about your antibiotic stewardship program is the best way to convey pertinent information about it to your prescribers.

4

DATA COLLECTION
AND THE PDCA CYCLE

A T THIS POINT, WE'VE SPENT A FAIR BIT OF TIME discussing the truth about antibiotics. We've talked about the three main culprits for inappropriate antibiotic use in long-term care facilities. And we've laid the foundation for an effective antibiotic stewardship program. Now it's time to turn our attention to the linchpin of every good antibiotic stewardship program: the data.

The best way to collect, measure, and report the right data is to enlist the help of your infection preventionist (IP). It makes sense when you think about it: Antibiotic stewardship and infection prevention go hand in hand. Indeed, you can't have good infection prevention and control (IPC) without antibiotic stewardship, and antibiotic stewardship without good IPC will never work. What's more, both IPC and antibiotic stewardship require proper data collection and reporting, so your IP should already have some familiarity with this essential task. However, chances are they will need to be properly trained to collect data that's actually meaningful to your stewardship program—and to report it in a way that compels action. We will dive into how to do that in this chapter.

YOUR IP IS YOUR MVP

Remember when we talked about the importance of only prescribing antibiotics when someone met the case definition for a suspected infection? A significant part of training the IP in data collection and reporting comes down to educating them on the McGeer criteria for UTIs, pneumonia, and pressure wound infections. By arming them with this information, you enable your IP to accurately determine what percentage of people were given antibiotics for infections they didn't actually have, which is crucial for moving the needle in your stewardship program. For instance, let's say that ten residents received antibiotics for presumed UTIs last month. If they understand the McGeer criteria for UTI, the IP could determine that only four of those people (for example) met the case definition—which means 60 percent of them received antibiotics for an infection they didn't have.

Once you've trained the IP on the McGeer criteria, provide them with a spreadsheet that makes it easy for them to collect all the relevant data. For your reference, here's an example of the presumed UTI spreadsheet I use when consulting at facilities. You can create similar spreadsheets for presumed pneumonia and presumed pressure wound infections (see the following page).

It's a good idea to cross-train someone else—the DON or the nurse educator, for example—on data collection as well, in case the IP goes on vacation, gets sick, or leaves.

COLLECT DATA DAILY

As you can see from the spreadsheet, all data should be collated on a monthly basis. However, the IP should collect the data daily. If they wait until the end of the month to do so, there is a high risk of the data being missed or recorded improperly. So train them to collect the data at each morning's stand-up meeting by asking which residents got cultures (or X-rays) and which were started on an antibiotic in the last twenty-four hours. Make sure they also find out what presumed infections those antibiotics were intended to treat. Then have them take that information back to their office, look at the notes and diagnostic results to determine whether or not the antibiotics and cultures were justified, and write that information down for later inclusion on the spreadsheet. Following this process will cut down on errors

ANTIBIOTIC STEWARDSHIP METRICS: THE FORUM
(Reporting Period) Worksheet

Metric	Initial Results	Month 1	Month 2	Month 3
Urine C&S orders				
Urine C&S positive				
Antibiotic Rx				
Rx with low colony count or multiple organisms				
Meeting standardized clinical criteria				
Antibiotic Rx empiric (before C&S result)				
Days of Antibiotic Therapy (DOT)				
C. difficile orders				
C. difficile positive				
ESBL+ urine isolates				

Definitions

Days of Therapy (DOT): Total number of days a patient is on any antibiotic. *Example*: Macrobid 100mg dispensed for 5 days would be 5 days of therapy (DOT) and 10 total doses.

Empiric Rx: Antibiotic Rx is started before culture results are known. Preferred strategy per stewardship protocol is use of 48-hour observation protocol in place of initiating empiric antibiotic Rx.

and, by making this a daily habit, your IP will never have to rush to complete their data collection and reporting for the monthly Q/A meeting.

EMPOWER YOUR IP TO ASK QUESTIONS

Your IP's training doesn't end with data collection. Remember in chapter 1 when I told you about Mary Matesan? One of the things that made her such a fantastic antibiotic steward was her willingness to question people about their actions. Whenever urine cultures were ordered, for example, Mary would ask why—and if a nurse or prescriber couldn't come up with a better reason than "the patient was confused," or "their urine was dark," she would read them the riot act. Train your IP to do the same. Empower them with information about the McGeer criteria for UTI, pneumonia, and pressure wound infection, and train them to be on the lookout for ASB masquerading as UTI, or a dry cough and an unknown infiltrate masquerading as pneumonia. If you do that, you'll create your own Mary Matesan—and believe me when I say your antibiotic stewardship program couldn't have a more valuable ally.

I know what you're probably thinking: "Our IP has a million things to do. They're not going to be happy about adding another task onto the rest of their responsibilities!" To that, I say: That's why cultivating interest and getting buy-in at the beginning is so important! Look, according to the CDC, over 35,000 people died from antibiotic-resistant infections in the United States in 2019.[15] Worldwide, more than 1.2 million died.[16]

Stop and take that in for a minute. We *must* start shifting how we do things, or those numbers will only get worse.

When your IP understands the problem—not just in their head, but deep in their heart—they'll be much more willing to do what it takes to solve it. And solving it, as you now know, requires your IP to collect, measure, and report the right data. It comes back to the truism I shared with you in the last chapter: *When you change the way you look at things, the things you look at change.* Get your IP to look at things differently, and it won't be long before what they're looking at—the data they're collecting and how they're collecting it—will change from focusing on how many pounds of antibiotics were used to far more meaningful information.

COLLECT BASELINE DATA

In the first quarter of your antibiotic stewardship program, all the IP needs to do is collect data by clinical syndrome (presumed

---

15 "National Infection & Death Estimates for Antimicrobial Resistance," Centers for Disease Control and Prevention, https://www.cdc.gov/drugresistance/national-estimates.html, accessed December 13, 2023.
16 "National Infection & Death Estimates."

UTI, presumed pneumonia, and presumed pressure wound infection) to establish a baseline for your facility. This allows everyone to see at a glance how often people received antibiotics for infections they didn't have. Remember, this data should be collected daily, collated monthly, and reported quarterly.

I know this is contrary to the type of data most facilities collect, so in case you still have some questions, let's dig into the process a little more. Every day at the stand-up meeting, as you know, the IP should collect information about how many antibiotics were given to people for presumed infections, and how many of those people actually met the case definition. Each month, they should compile that information into the report spreadsheet (see the example above). Then, at the end of the quarter, the IP should put together a report that summarizes their findings.

For example, the report might state, "In month one, we gave antibiotics to ninety people for a presumed urinary tract infection. Ten of them met the case definition. The rest of them had asymptomatic bacteriuria that was misidentified as UTI. In month two, we gave antibiotics to eighty-six people for presumed UTI; eleven of them met the case definition. In month three, we gave antibiotics to eighty people for presumed UTI. Seven of them met the case definition."

That report will then go to the medical director. Once the director reviews it, they should draft a letter explaining the findings. The letter should also establish a goal for the next quarter. The goal might be to decrease empiric use of antibiotics, reduce the number of cultures, or (more specifically) reduce the number of antibiotics given for ASB or misdiagnosed pneumonia. After signing the letter, they should send it to each of the facility's prescribers so they can see where the facility stands. Sending the information on to the prescribers also supports the expectations first set in the announcement letter—namely, that empiric antibiotic use in the facility is no longer the name of the game. The following quarter, the whole cycle starts over again and continues on and on into perpetuity. *A note here: When you start collecting data, don't be surprised if the numbers are (to put it mildly) shocking.*

I've consulted for facilities that have put thirty patients on antibiotics in a month, even though none of them met the case definition for the suspected infection. And as the following graphic shows, I've also seen facilities where cultures were ordered for more than fifty people in a month. Twenty-four of them were put on antibiotics, and yet only one of those people met the case definition for infection.

Remember, antibiotics are deeply entrenched in our culture; sometimes, seeing numbers like that is what it takes to wake people up.

ANTIBIOTIC STEWARDSHIP METRICS
First Quarterly Report 2015

Metric	Results
Urine C&S orders	56
Urine C&S positive	39
Antibiotic Rx	24
Rx with low colony count	10
Meeting standardized clinical criteria	1
Days of Antibiotic Therapy (DOT)	186
Antibiotic Rx—empiric	TBA
C. difficile orders	10
C. difficile positive	2

THE PDCA CYCLE

Collecting, measuring, and reporting on a quarterly cycle helps filter out the noise of natural variations by focusing on trends over time. Reporting more frequently, on the other hand, introduces the very real possibility that people will react to individual numbers rather than trends. We've all experienced this—I call it *data insanity*. Let's say that one month, 64 percent of patients receive antibiotics for infections they don't have. The next month, 62.5 percent receive antibiotics. If you were looking at month-over-month data, that seeming 1.5 percent reduction might be cause for celebration. But then, the next month, maybe it jumps back up to 64 percent. Because you were reporting monthly, you celebrated too early.

The moral of the story? Look at trends based on a quarterly cycle: I promise, it will give you far more accurate insights into what's going on at your facility.

Collecting and measuring data in this way follows what's known as the PDCA (Plan-Do-Check-Act) cycle. This model focuses on a continuous loop of planning (determining the goals for a process and the changes necessary to achieve them), doing (implementing the changes), checking (evaluating the results), and acting (stabilizing the change or, if necessary, beginning the cycle again).

In this instance, the *plan* is to reduce the overuse of antibiotics by decreasing empiric antibiotic use. The prescribers are expected to *implement* this change by only prescribing antibiotics when a patient meets the case definition for a given infection. The IP *evaluates* the results by collecting the appropriate data. If inappropriate antibiotic use decreases, great! If not, the PDCA cycle *starts again*.

It's very rare that any facility moves the needle forward significantly in the first quarter or two. Usually, it takes several iterations before noticeable results are achieved. And you know what? That's okay! In my experience, the best experiments are the ones that *don't* work. That's the beauty of the PDCA cycle: it allows for continuous improvement. Get a result you don't like? Review the data and try something a little different. Then, next quarter, check the data again. Keep refining and tweaking until your results are where you want them.

Stay with it, and you'll begin seeing results within a few quarters. The number of cultures and X-rays ordered will decrease. The number of patients treated with low colony count will decrease. Total days of therapy will go down. The number of patients who don't meet the case definition for an infection but receive antibiotics anyway will be reduced. And eventually, antibiotic resistance will begin to unwind.

BREAK THE HYPNOSIS

Engaging in the PDCA cycle (and, of course, making sure your IP is collecting, measuring, and reporting data accurately and consistently) will help break the "hypnosis" so many pre-scribers are under of reflexively prescribing antibiotics even when a patient doesn't meet the strict case definition for an infection. It's a way to change the way they look at things so that the things they look at change. And that, it bears repeating, is the goal.

To keep the cycle going, make it a point to celebrate prog-ress every six months or so. Acknowledge all the successes that have occurred, and take some time to recognize every-one who played a role in bringing those achievements to life.

Make the celebration public, too. For example, you could put posters up in the facility honoring your entire team, or hold an awards luncheon for all the prescribers and staff who worked so hard to move the needle for you.

If there are failures (and there will be from time to time), make an effort to figure out why things went wrong, then fix them. Once you've turned a failure into a success, celebrate that, too. Of course, the old saying holds true here: You don't have to air your dirty laundry in public. But that doesn't mean you should shy away from failure, either. Remember that it's often the best way to course-correct and create wins that can be celebrated.

THE SEVEN CORE ELEMENTS OF GOOD STEWARDSHIP

At this point in the program, chances are high that you understand *why* you should implement a strong antibiotic stewardship program. You also have a basic idea of how to get one started (although we'll dive into some of the nuances of a good program later in the book). But if you're like many of the people I talk to, you're probably experiencing some trepidation. You've probably read through the core elements that the CDC published about antibiotic stewardship, but they weren't particularly straightforward or accessible, right? So now you're wondering: does the protocol I've laid out over the last few chapters meet all CDC and CMS requirements?

Great question! In a nutshell, the answer is yes. The antibiotic stewardship protocol is designed to promote optimal use of antibiotics and to assist facilities to meet CMS requirements. As a result, it corresponds neatly to the seven CDC core elements of antibiotic stewardship in nursing homes.[17]

To show you how, let's go through each core element one by one and compare it to the corresponding element in the antibiotic stewardship program I've laid out for you.

The CDC's first core element is **leadership commitment**. By this, the CDC means that nursing home leaders must commit to improving antibiotic use. Think back to the first steps in the protocol: scheduling and holding the senior team meeting. This meeting, which includes (at a minimum) the administrator, the director of nursing, the medical director, and the infection preventionist, ensures aligned commitment. Not only that, but the announcement letter that should come out of this meeting notifies everyone of leadership's support for the program.

The second element is **accountability**. With this element, the CDC wants to see that the administration engages and holds the medical director, director of nursing, consulting pharmacist,

---

17 "Core Elements of Antibiotic Stewardship for Nursing Homes," Centers for Disease Control and Prevention, https://www.cdc.gov/antibiotic-use/core-elements/nursing-homes.html, accessed January 19, 2024.

and infection preventionist accountable. When you follow the protocol I've laid out, this is exactly what happens. The senior leadership team, particularly the medical director, supports the stewardship program and authors all communications and reports, which means in essence that everyone is held accountable to adhering to proper antibiotic use.

The third element is **drug expertise**. This element establishes access to individuals with antibiotic expertise. The protocol covers this element by including consulting pharmacists in the program's team.

Fourth is **action**. The CDC and CMS want to see that policy and practice changes improve antibiotic use. The protocol adheres to this element by actively monitoring antibiotic prescribing and reviewing quarterly summary metrics. Taken in tandem, this fosters appropriate prescribing practices.

Fifth, we have **tracking**. This element requires facilities to monitor antibiotic use practices and outcomes to guide interventions. When you follow the program I've laid out, you achieve this by collecting metrics (such as days of therapy) to measure both frequency and appropriateness of culturing and antibiotic prescriptions.

Sixth is **reporting**. The CDC wants to see that facilities report outcomes, adverse events, and costs from antibiotics. Sounds daunting, right? But once again, my program has you covered. When you follow it, sequential quarterly summary

CROSS-WALK
CDC Core Elements vs. Antibiotic Stewardship Protocol Features

CDC Core Element	Stewardship Protocol Feature
Leadership Commitment: Nursing home leaders commit to improving antibiotic use.	Meeting of senior team (admin, DON, medical director, IP) ensures aligned commitment. Announcement letter notifies all of program intent.
Accountability: Administration engages and holds accountable the medical director, DON, consulting pharmacist, and infection preventionist.	Facility medical director supports stewardship program and authors all communications and reports.
Drug Expertise: Establishes access to individuals with antibiotic expertise.	Consulting pharmacists are included in each facility program team.
Action: Policy and practice changes improve antibiotic use.	Active prescribing surveillance and quarterly summary metrics foster appropriate prescribing practices.
Tracking: Monitoring antibiotic use practices and outcomes guides interventions.	Report metrics (days of therapy, etc.) measure frequency and appropriateness of culturing and antibiotic Rx.
Reporting: outcomes, adverse events, and costs from antibiotics.	Sequential quarterly summary reports are discussed at facility QA committee and distributed to all prescribers by medical director.
Education: Provide resources to prescribers, nurses, residents, and families about antibiotic resistance and improving use.	In-services addressing new standards of practice are provided for nurses, prescribers, and families.

Interpretive Note: The Antibiotic Stewardship protocol is designed to promote optimal use of antibiotics and to assist client facilities to meet new CMS requirements. The facility medical director is positioned to lead the program, and all communications and reports go out over his/her signature. The stewardship program effectively maps onto the recently released seven (7) CDC Core Elements of Antibiotic Stewardship in Nursing Homes—see above.

reports are discussed by the Q/A committee and distributed to all prescribers by the medical director.

The final core element is **education**. The CDC expects facilities to provide resources to prescribers, nurses, residents, and families about antibiotic resistance and improving use. Using the resources I've shared with you in this book, you can educate nurses, prescribers, residents, and their families about new standards of practice in a variety of forums.

So there you have it: the basic steps to implementing an effective antibiotic stewardship program. Remember to cultivate interest first so you can get buy-in from your entire staff. Once you've done that, it's time to start training your residents and their families, your nurses and CNAs, and your prescribers in the fine art of reducing inappropriate antibiotic use. Spend time training your IP to collect, measure, and report on the data as well, and enlist the medical director to communicate those findings to the prescribers. Finally, utilize the PDCA cycle to foster continuous improvement, and celebrate your wins and successes regularly to keep spirits and engagement high.

KEY TAKEAWAYS

- Your IP is uniquely situated to collect the proper data about the effectiveness of your antibiotic stewardship program.

- Make sure your IP has the right tools and the right training to collect the right data.
- Following the PDCA cycle will give your stewardship program the best chance of success.
- Celebrate successes regularly to keep your staff engaged and excited about the stewardship program.
- Follow the antibiotic stewardship protocol I've laid out to ensure compliance with the CDC's seven core elements of antibiotic stewardship in nursing homes.

5

MDROs AND ANTIBIOTIC STEWARDSHIP

S O OFTEN AFTER I TELL PEOPLE THE TRUTH ABOUT antibiotics, I see them nodding in agreement. Most people have at least heard that antibiotics are widely overused, and (to some extent, anyway) they know that overuse can lead to some negative outcomes. Despite this knowledge, though, when the rubber meets the road, far too many people—patients and doctors alike—reach for antibiotics anytime they're faced with the smallest sign of illness.

This is especially true in nursing home settings. Resident has a viral infection? Antibiotics can't possibly help you beat it, but many times, the resident or their family demand an antibiotic anyway. Resident "just knows" they have a UTI? No problem, they think: antibiotics to the rescue! Prescribers justify it to themselves by thinking something like, "Well, if I prescribe an antibiotic, it will prevent a supervening bacterial infection." And then they write the prescription, and on they go to the next patient, where— nine times out of ten—the same scenario will play out all over again.

Cue the violins, because this ship is going down.

I don't want to beat a dead horse, but like the *Titanic*, we're charging full speed ahead at the iceberg of inappropriately prescribed antibiotics. The only difference is that, unlike that ill-fated ship, we still have time to course-correct. But we need to do it now.

Things aren't all doom and gloom, though. If we can change course—and for the purposes of this book, that simply means getting nurses and prescribers and residents to start changing how they think about antibiotics—antibiotic resistance will unwind, and it will do so fast. Remember the illustration I showed you way back in chapter 1? To save you having to flip back to it, here it is again:

180-Bed SNF Stewardship Results 2015

Metric	4Q 2014	1Q 2015	2Q 2015	3Q 2015	4Q 2015	
Urine C&S orders	94	63	26	27	21	←
Urine C&S positive	65	46	12	16	10	
Days of UTI Antibiotic Therapy		268			85	
C. difficile orders	12	15	6	3	9	
C. difficile positive	7	4	4	0	0	←
ESBL + urine isolates	21	7	4	4	4	←

This is a perfect illustration of how quickly change can occur. Just look at the numbers! Within a year, the number of *C. diff* infections went from seven to zero. (I'll be honest—that was a surprise, because we didn't expect to see such incredible results so quickly. And yet, the data doesn't lie.) The number of ESBL positive organisms, a marker of resistance, also dropped quite quickly, from twenty-one to only four.

Why? Because the only thing that's holding multiple resistance in place is the obscene overuse of antibiotics. It's that pressure, and *nothing* else, that's at the root of resistance. If you removed that pressure from your own facility overnight, you'd see results just like this within the first month. That's why this work is so important: We think of antibiotic resistance as a global problem (and it is), but it's one that can be solved at the local level, facility by facility, and community by community.

In other words, don't wait for the entire world to start doing this work. Let it start at home, with me and thee.

MULTIDRUG-RESISTANT ORGANISMS (MDROs)

Of course, with all this talk about resistance, we've got to spend some time talking about the elephant in the room: MDROs, or multidrug-resistant organisms. I know I'm sticking my neck out here because this is such a controversial topic, but I vowed long ago that I was going to speak the truth. So hold your nose, because we're jumping in.

Broadly speaking, the emergence of MDROs is related to antibiotic usage. But how do you address MDROs in the short term and long term? Let's examine the answer to that question using MRSA (methicillin-resistant staph aureus) as an example. You see, even though it doesn't incite the same level of panic that it used to, MRSA is still a problem, especially in long-term care facilities. If you culture someone and it comes back that they have MRSA, chances are high that person will get put in isolation. That presents a problem, though, doesn't it? On the one hand, the CDC wants facilities to follow isolation guidelines. On the other hand, they don't want facilities to interfere with the patient's right to socialize.

No conflict there, right? (And yes, I just rolled my eyes.)

Luckily for our MRSA patient, there's a better way to approach things: Instead of isolation precautions, you can use decolonization procedures. A study[18] published in *The New England Journal of Medicine* describes the protocol: Use chlorhexidine for all routine bathing and showering, and administer nasal povidone-iodine twice daily for the first five days and then twice daily for five days every other week. When this protocol is followed, there is a significantly lower risk that residents with MRSA (and other MDROs) will need to be transferred to a hospital due to infection than if you provided routine care.

Standard isolation procedures are, if I'm being blunt, cruelty masquerading as effective action. To make things even worse, there's actually very little evidence that isolation measures make any significant difference. They're put in place to reduce the spread of MRSA (or any other MDRO) to other residents. However, in and of themselves, isolation procedures don't help people who have an MDRO get better.

That's a problem. According to the CDC, over 3 million antimicrobial-resistant infections occur each year in the United States alone, and more than 48,000 people die as a result.[19]

---

18   Loren G. Miller et al., "Decolonization in Nursing Homes to Prevent Infection and Hospitalization," *New England Journal of Medicine* 389, no. 19 (October 10, 2023): 1766–77. https://www.nejm.org/doi/full/10.1056/NEJMoa2215254.

19   "2019 AR Threats Report," Centers for Disease Control and Prevention, https://www.cdc.gov/drugresistance/biggest-threats.html, accessed March 14, 2024.

And residents in long-term care facilities face a disproportionate threat, because they live in a congregate setting and often have multiple comorbidities. However, by using decolonization measures *and* continuing with a strong antibiotic stewardship program, you can decrease MDROs like MRSA among your population. Combining these two approaches ensures that residents in the facility are helped in the short term through decolonization procedures. In the long term, antibiotic resistance is reduced or eliminated because the radical overuse of unnecessary antibiotics is stopped.

C. *DIFF* AND ANTIBIOTIC OVERUSE

Along with other types of multidrug resistance, antibiotic overuse leads to *C. diff*. In fact, if you go back in time, you'll see that almost 90 percent of *C. diff* cases have a history of antibiotic therapy in the previous three months. And here's another little fun fact that will make you scratch your head: It's the only disease I can think of that is both caused by and traditionally treated with antibiotics.

C. diff is the bane of nursing homes, both because it can spread through the resident population like wildfire and because, historically, it's been incredibly difficult to treat. However, the Mayo Clinic in Phoenix has been able to successfully treat it with fecal transplants. I won't get into the specifics of how they work (although if you're interested, you can find out more by watching the video referenced in the corresponding footnote[20]). However, in most cases, within forty-eight hours after receiving a transplant, patients walk out of the hospital completely cured. It's pretty incredible, and perhaps best of all, *no antibiotics are used in treatment*. In my experience, once people have gone through C. *diff* and come out the other side, they've seen the light. Come hell or high water, they don't want to mess with inappropriate antibiotics ever again. But let's not wait for residents to get C. *diff* before stopping empirical prescribing, okay? Let's make the change now.

DEALING WITH C. AURIS

C. auris. In the old days, the running joke at my microbiology lab went like this: "How do you scare the living daylights out of a nurse? Call her and say, 'The blood culture shows *Acinetobacter calcoaceticus* variant *lwoffii*.'" Nowadays, though, if you want to terrify a nurse, all you have to do is call and say, "Yes, I'm from the laboratory, and we're growing *Candida auris* in the urine from Mrs. Jones." That little bug is worse than Freddy Krueger on Elm Street, I'm telling you.

20 Mayo Clinic, "Fecal Transplant to Treat C. Difficile Infection - Sahil Khanna, MBBS - Mayo Clinic," May 7, 2013, YouTube video, 2:58,https://www.youtube.com/watch?v=A5ONGXnNp4U.

As soon as nurses hear *C. auris*, they start thinking about isolation procedures. They think about scrubbing down the whole facility. Bringing in the biohazard guys in their hazmat suits. Spraying *everything*. Suddenly, their day is looking really, really bleak.

Maybe I shouldn't be flippant. I understand that *C. auris* is a big deal. In fact, I debated whether or not to even mention it here. But when it comes to MDROs, *C. auris* is the elephant in the room, and I didn't want to leave you hanging. And I won't: Decolonization procedures have been shown to be effective against organisms like *C. auris*, too. In fact, decolonization can help against any of the organisms that the CDC has identified as urgent, serious, and concerning.[21,22] And remember, when you couple short-term decolonization procedures with a strong antibiotic stewardship program, resistance will begin to rapidly unwind, and pretty soon, these MDROs will be a thing of the past.

ENHANCED BARRIER PRECAUTIONS

Many times, when I talk to facilities about MDROs, they ask me about enhanced barrier precautions. Obviously, they are better for residents than standard contact isolation procedures.

---

21 "2019 AR Threats Report."
22 Miller et al., "Decolonization in Nursing Homes."

However, I think that decolonization makes more sense. When you decolonize people, you get rid of the MDRO and remove any temptation to use antibiotics to treat people. Remember, neither isolation procedures nor enhanced barrier precautions can cure a person infected with a multidrug-resistant organism. Those procedures are in place simply to keep other people safe. Decolonizing eliminates the MDRO so it's no longer a threat to the infected person or the people around them.

IT'S ALL ABOUT THE POLICY

Of course, I'm not naive. Even though decolonization makes a lot of sense, it flies in the face of what the CDC advises. Not only that, but every long-term care facility has to face the very real fact that CMS surveyors are going to come in and, if everything isn't just so, potentially issue citations or even IJs. For that reason, it's natural to worry about following decolonization procedures rather than isolation procedures.

That's why I tell every facility I consult for that it's all about the policy. When it comes to determining whether you're in compliance with protocol or not, a good surveyor will ask you one simple question: "What does your policy say?" If you have a policy in place that clearly maps out what you should do when someone has an MDRO, *and* you follow it, then you should be fine.

Let me say it another way: *You can dare to be innovative and leading-edge rather than blindly adhering to mindless protocols as long as you have a good policy in place and you follow that policy to a T.* The bottom line is that surveyors aren't in the business of critiquing policy.

Of course, you need to be smart about it. There's a whole chain of things you need to do to make sure that when a surveyor asks if you're following the policy, you can say yes. Often, it comes down to training. Does every single member of your staff know your policies? Does every single member of your staff adhere to them? What about the housekeepers? The brand-new CNA that just came onboard? The nurse who has been at your facility for twenty years and likes to do things "the way they've always been done"? Just like with your antibiotic stewardship program, you need to make sure that everyone is on notice about your MDRO policies. They should be able to explain their role in upholding them, and they should follow them to the letter, 100 percent of the time.

HOW TO WRITE A POLICY

With all this talk of policies, it makes sense to spend a little time unpacking how to write a good one. There are obviously many ways to write a policy, and every facility has its own way. However, there are some basic things every good policy should include, as the illustration below shows:

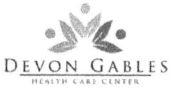

DEVON GABLES HEALTH CARE CENTER
Policy Title
Rev 1.0
Revision Date: | Effective Date: 5/10/2023

1. Purpose
   1.1.

2. Scope
   2.1.

3. Policy
   3.1.

4. Implementation
   4.1.

5. Procedure
   5.1.

6. References and Related Documents
   6.1.

7. Revision History
   7.1. *Document Creation/Approval*

	Name	Signature	Position	Date
Prepared by	Jane Anderson		Director of Nursing	
Approved by	Dr. John Smith		Medical Director	

   7.2. *Revision Review*

New Revision Number	Revisions Made	Made By	Approved By	Effective Date

   7.3. *Annual Review*

	Year	Name	Signature	Position	Date
Reviewed by					
Reviewed by					
Reviewed by					
Reviewed by					

Of course, not every policy has to incorporate these exact headings. Do what makes sense for what you're talking about. For instance, here is an example of a policy I put together for implementing antibiotic stewardship programs (and yes, you should have a similar policy based on the protocol I shared with you—you're welcome!):

SAMPLE

Section: Infection Prevention and Control
Subject: Policy For Antibiotic Stewardship Program
Effective Date: ... 2024

Background

Antibiotic resistance is now considered one of the most urgent national and global public health threats. Antibiotic use is receiving considerable national attention. Diseases caused by multidrug-resistant bacteria are increasing in long-term care facilities and contributing to higher rates of morbidity and mortality. Under the SNF proposed rules changes, post-acute and long-term care facilities will be mandated by CMS to regularly review antibiotic utilization and to have programs in place to promote optimal prescribing practices. <facility name> is now implementing a practical antibiotic stewardship protocol, now available as an implementation-ready package. This policy is aligned with the CDC Core Elements of Antibiotic Stewardship for Nursing Homes.[23]

Policy

It is the policy of <facility name> to implement an Antibiotic Stewardship Program (ASP) which will promote appropriate use of antibiotics while optimizing the treatment of infections, and at the same time reducing the adverse events associated with antibiotic use. This policy is intended to limit antibiotic resistance in the post-acute care setting while improving treatment efficacy and resident safety and reducing treatment-related costs.

ASP activities in post-acute facilities include these basic elements: leadership commitment, accountability, drug expertise, action to implement recommended policies or practices, tracking measures, reporting data, and education for clinicians, nursing staff, residents, and families about antibiotic resistance and opportunities for improvement.

23 "Core Elements of Antibiotic Stewardship for Nursing Homes."

Procedure

1. Leadership commitment
   a. The senior leadership of <facility name> is committed to supporting the safe and appropriate use of antibiotics.
      i. The medical director will communicate the facility's expectations for antibiotic use to prescribing clinicians.
   b. ASP champions within facility staff will be identified and supported.
2. Accountability
   a. An ASP Team will be established to be accountable for stewardship activities. The ASP Team will consist of the medical director, administrator, director of nursing (DON), infection preventionist (IP), MDS coordinator, and pharmacy consultant. As a team they will:
      i. Review infections and monitor antibiotic usage patterns on a regular basis
      ii. Obtain and review antibiograms for institutional trends of resistance
      iii. Monitor multidrug-resistant organisms (MRSA, VRE, ESBL, CRE, etc.) and *Clostridium difficile* infections.

        iv. Report monthly or quarterly, as appropriate, the number of antibiotics prescribed (e.g., days of therapy) and other standardized metrics per protocol.

        v. Include a separate report section for the number of residents on antibiotics that did not meet criteria for active infection.

    b. Microbiology laboratory provider will submit a facility-specific antibiogram on a regular basis, e.g. annually.

    c. Facility will designate who will collect and review antibiotic surveillance data.

3. Drug Expertise

    a. Pharmacy consultant will be engaged to review and make written recommendations on antibiotic usage patterns.

    b. Facility may consider retaining an infectious-disease-trained physician or pharmacist to provide additional guidance to the ASP Team for developing new methods for working with prescribers and residents' families.

4. Action

    a. The antibiotic stewardship protocol will address:

        i. Root cause of widespread antibiotic resistance.

      ii. Focused improvement response aimed at altering outmoded prescribing habits.

      iii. Auditing antibiotic usage as related to specific clinical syndromes, e.g. urinary tract infection.

      iv. Structured feedback to prescribers and nurses directed toward facilitating a transition in thinking.

      v. New approach to common urinary tract scenarios as an alternative to empiric antibiotic Rx in low-likelihood scenarios, e.g. forty-eight-hour observation pathway.

  b. A method of identifying and tracking residents with multidrug-resistant organisms (MDROs) will be established.

5. Tracking

  a. IP will be responsible for infection surveillance and MDRO tracking.

  b. IP will collect and report data per protocol such as:

      i. Number of positive cultures.

      ii. Number of patients with positive cultures who were treated with an antibiotic.

iii. Number of patients treated with antibiotics who meet McGeer criteria for active infection.

iv. Number of post-antibiotic complications, e.g. *Clostridium difficile* infections.

c. Pharmacy consultant will review and report antibiotic usage patterns, most specifically recommendations made to prescribers as follow-up to quarterly stewardship protocol reporting.

6. Reporting

a. IP and/or other members of the ASP Team will review and report findings to facility staff and to the quality assurance/QAPI committee, who will then provide feedback to facility staff.

b. Feedback will be given by the medical director to prescribers on their individual laboratory ordering practices and prescribing patterns, as indicated.

7. Education

a. Educational opportunities on the appropriate use of antibiotics, as identified by the ASP Team, will be provided at regular intervals for clinical staff as well as residents and their families.

No matter what headings you include or how you set them up, make sure each of your policies includes a signature at the end indicating who wrote and authorized it. Usually, policies are signed by the manager and medical director. Every year, the policy should be reviewed and, if necessary, updated.

Since CDC and CMS regulations require facilities to have antibiotic stewardship programs, make sure you have a policy that lays out exactly what your program looks like. Specifically, your policy should highlight the three main culprits for inappropriate antibiotic use (presumed UTI, pneumonia, and pressure wound infections) and how everyone at your facility will handle each of them. Make sure your policy includes information about how you will collect and report data, too.

Best practice when it comes to antibiotic stewardship policies is to also include language explaining that everybody in a position key to the success of the program should have a backup. In other words, the policy should outline who will cover for each role and provide for cross-training for relevant personnel. That way, if your facility is short-staffed for any reason, your program won't get disrupted or thrown off course.

Now that you have a good understanding of how to handle instances of MDROs that come up while you're implementing your antibiotic stewardship program—not to mention how to write a strong policy that will satisfy even the most diligent CMS surveyor—let's turn our attention to some case studies. The idea behind sharing these studies is to give you real-world examples and information about what's possible when you implement the antibiotic stewardship protocol I've described. Whether you have a single small facility, a large campus, or a network of multiple facilities, you'll see what a difference this stewardship program can make. Even better, you'll understand some of the potential pitfalls you might encounter and how to avoid them. Ready? Me too. Onward and upward!

KEY TAKEAWAYS

- Broadly speaking, the emergence of MDROs is related to antibiotic usage.
- Rather than utilizing isolation precautions, consider using decolonization procedures to address MDROs like MRSA.
- To avoid citations and IJs from CMS surveyors, make sure you have policies in place clearly outlining how your facility handles MDROs.
- Train every member of your staff thoroughly on your policies, and ensure they adhere to them 100 percent of the time.

- When you write a policy, make sure it includes, at minimum, the purpose, scope, policy description, implementation, procedure, references and related documents, and revision history information. It should also include an area for signatures and dates reviewed.

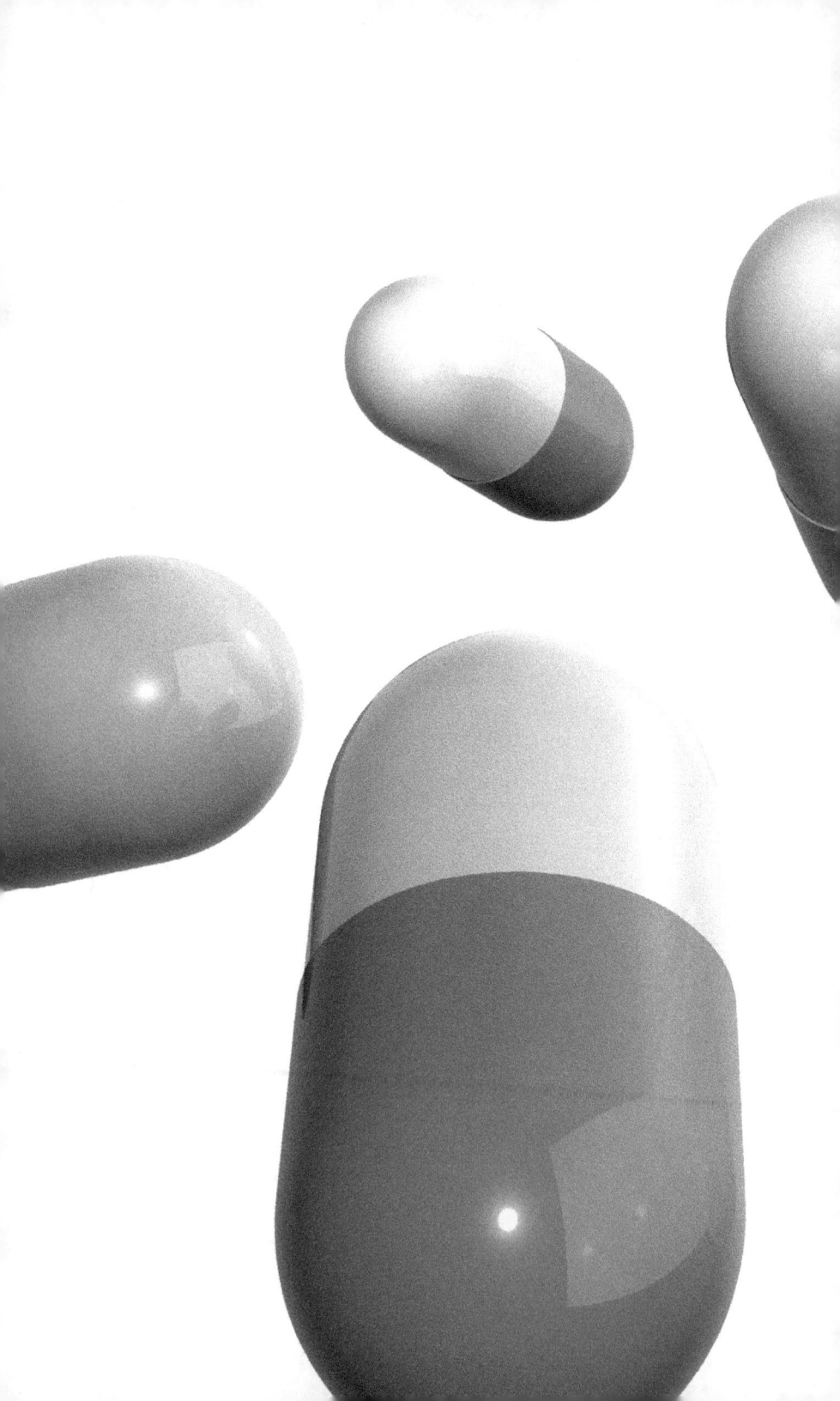

PART 3

CASE
STUDIES

N ow that you have a good understanding of what goes into building and maintaining an effective antibiotic stewardship program, it's time to round out your knowledge with real-world examples. I've chosen three different case studies from facilities I've worked with to share with you here.

The first, Devon Gables, was chosen because it highlights the latest best practices I've come up with based on my years of doing this work. We launched Devon Gables' revival program late in 2023, so as of this writing, we are very much at the beginning of the program. That's exciting, though, because it offers an opportunity for me to share some of the most important components of getting a program up and running with you. Whether you're reviving an old antibiotic stewardship program that fell by the wayside (perhaps because of the pandemic) or starting a program from scratch, there are lessons to be learned from following the start of Devon Gables' journey.

The second case study looks more closely at the antibiotic stewardship program in a facility I've mentioned previously: Glencroft. This was one of the most successful stewardship programs I've ever seen, and I'm looking forward to diving into what specifically made the program so effective. My hope is that, after you read the chapter about Glencroft, you'll be far better equipped to mimic the conditions that led to its success in your own facility.

Finally, we'll take a look at a unique scenario: implementing an antibiotic stewardship program from the ground up for Covenant Health Network, which is a multistate, multinetwork operation. It was a huge undertaking—we were focusing on building the program for not one, not two, but eleven facilities all at once. While we made good progress, there were some challenges that barred us from achieving the kind of success I was hoping for. However, hindsight is 20/20, as they say, and I learned a lot from the experience. Whether you're part of a network or involved with a single facility, I think you'll be able to learn a lot through this case study, too. Even more importantly, the lessons I share with you in that chapter will help you avoid making the same mistakes in your program that we did in Covenant's program.

So what do you say...ready to dive into the case studies? Then let's get to it!

6

DEVON GABLES

F OR THE FIRST PART OF MY CAREER, I WORKED "behind the microscope" in a pathology laboratory. I lived in Arizona then (as I do now), and I would spend two weeks at a time working in a lab in Yuma, then head up to a little gambling town in northwestern Arizona to work for the alternate two weeks. It was a grueling cycle, going back and forth between those two labs and my home in Phoenix every few weeks. I enjoyed it, but eventually, I had to face facts: I was exhausted. Living out of a suitcase was quickly losing its appeal.

Just about the time I was ready to get out of that game, I saw an ad in a local pathology newsletter. It was for a medical director position at Diagnostic Labs and Radiology, a mobile diagnostics company that traveled to nursing homes to perform X-rays and lab services. The position looked amazing: I would be home every night, but I could still work in pathology. I applied and got the job.

I was forty-five years old, but my real career—and, it turned out, my life's work in antibiotic stewardship—was just beginning. Pretty soon, I had moved beyond the scope of responsibilities outlined by the ad. I was spending a large chunk of time helping our salespeople answer client questions and talk them down when they were upset about something. Before long, I became the go-to guy for that, because people knew I could listen to just about anybody and speak reasonably with them.

It was around that same time that I started talking with everyone who would listen about antibiotic stewardship. My time in the lab drove home the importance of reducing inappropriate antibiotic prescribing, and I shouted that truth from every rooftop I could. It wasn't long before I was more than just the go-to guy for upset clients or people with questions; I was the go-to guy for antibiotic stewardship.

Eventually, I moved on from Diagnostic Labs and Radiology, but my reputation as an antibiotic stewardship expert remained. I met lots of great people who supported the work, one of whom I'm excited to tell you about in this chapter: John Wadleigh, D.O.

Dr. Wadleigh was one of the people with whom I had spent so much time talking about antibiotic stewardship. Clearly, I made an impression: Some years back, he and I ended up attending the same national conference. We were in a room full of people—at least 100, maybe more. The topic? You guessed it: antibiotic stewardship. Not long into the presentation, I felt a gentle tap on my shoulder. Turning around, I saw Dr. Wadleigh. "You should be up there doing all this," he said to me. "The people up there are a bunch of academics who don't know shit from Shinola when it comes to this stuff!"

Strong language, perhaps, but it made me laugh. It also made me think. The people on the panel that day were talking a lot about stewardship, yes, but like so many other so-called experts, they weren't telling the truth about antibiotics. Instead, they were saying things like, "Well, you know, sometimes some prescribers overuse antibiotics." Dr. Wadleigh was right: I've been in this game for years, and I've learned that wimpy comments like that don't create meaningful change. That's why I tell the truth—that the main problem in infectious disease today is people receiving antibiotics for infections they do not have, and that the root cause of the resistance problems we see today is the overuse of antibiotics—and I do it like the hammer of Thor. Dr. Wadleigh knew that, which is why he said I should have been leading the discussion that day.

STARTING THE POST-COVID REVIVAL

Fast forward to 2023. I was ready to expand my antibiotic stewardship protocol to more facilities and was thinking about which might make good candidates. Having known Dr. Wadleigh for such a long time, his name immediately sprang to mind.

Dr. Wadleigh is the medical director at Devon Gables, a large (300+ beds) skilled nursing community that offers rehabilitation care, long-term care, Alzheimer's services, assisted living, and independent living options. Needless to say, it's a big operation with a lot going on!

Like so many other facilities, their antibiotic stewardship program was hit hard by the pandemic. However, prior to COVID-19, they had been committed to reducing antibiotic overuse in their facility. So I decided to take a chance and give Dr. Wadleigh a call.

I remember when he picked up the phone. I said, "Hey, Dr. Wadleigh, I'm a voice from your past." There was a pause, and then, with a smile in his voice, he said, "It's really good to hear from you, Dr. Patterson! You know, we have a lot of history together, don't we?" And we do—all of it good, and most of it centered around the work I've done with antibiotic stewardship.

After we caught up for a few minutes, I told him why I was calling. "I want to help you get your antibiotic stewardship program back up and running," I said. "What days of the week are you at Devon Gables?" He immediately responded with something that made my heart sing: "I'm there on Mondays and Thursdays, but why don't you come on a Monday because that's when I meet with my nurse practitioners. You can come to one of those meetings so you can talk to them, too."

Bingo! I was in.

When I arrived at Devon Gables, I realized they had spent almost a year trying to get their program back up and running. And here's the thing: They had done a decent job, but their program wasn't as effective as it could have been. That's why I'm so excited to share what we did with you. If you're in the same boat, you will be able to see how the theory of the protocol that I shared with you earlier can play out in practice, especially if you commit to it wholeheartedly like the leadership and staff at Devon Gables have done.

PRIORITIZING THE IN-SERVICE DAYS

The first step to getting Devon Gables' program turned around, of course, was to meet with the leadership team and get the announcement letter written. I have a template for this letter (which I shared with you earlier), so I had the letter in hand during the meeting. Along with Dr. Wadleigh, I met with Janelle Levitt (DON), Heather Friebus (administrator), and Maricela Nuñez (infection preventionist). I have a long history with Heather, too, so it was great fun to be able to work with her again.

I opened with them the way I suggest you do with your own leadership team: with a blunt discussion of the truth about antibiotic overuse and the disastrous consequences we face if we don't start making changes now. I was in luck; they are a great team of people, and they understood my point almost immediately. They signed the letter, and we were off to the races.

Once the senior team was on board, I worked with Maricela to coordinate the next step—convincing the staff to jump on the stewardship bandwagon. I already had leadership's blessing; now I just needed to get staff buy-in. The best way to do that (and the same will be true for you at your facility) was to bring everyone together and do the whole dog and pony show all over again.

We decided to start with the nurse practitioners, because it was important to get the prescribers on board. So at 8:00 a.m. on the Monday following the senior team meeting, I met with the NPs. Dr. Wadleigh introduced me to them as the antibiotic stewardship expert, which made my job a whole lot easier. There were six NPs present, and as I talked to them, I was watching their faces to see how my words landed. It will be important for you to do this, too, because you want to catch any potential resistance or obstacles as soon as possible so you can address them before they end up potentially sinking the whole ship.

The only pushback we received was from one NP who was worried about sepsis. She'd had a patient, it turns out, who had asymptomatic bacteriuria and then got urinary sepsis and had to go to the hospital. I listened, and then reassured her that the UTI protocol I suggest using (the one I shared with you earlier in the book) recommends monitoring patients closely for any change in condition while you're pushing fluids. If any signs of urinary sepsis appear, then it's important to get that person to the hospital and onto a sepsis protocol immediately. However, those instances are rare and certainly don't warrant indiscriminately passing out antibiotics every time a patient has "smelly" urine or seems a bit confused. I reminded her, and I'll remind you now, that a good antibiotic stewardship program isn't about eliminating antibiotics. It's about eliminating "just in case" antibiotics. There's a big difference.

After I spoke with the NPs, Maricela and I set up a time to talk to the rest of the staff. I spent the whole day speaking with dozens of personnel about what we were trying to accomplish, why it was important, and what their role in it would be. That first in-service day—which was a rousing success—laid the foundation for the education portion of the program that I shared with you in part 2.

As you conduct your own education and training, keep the story about the NP's resistance in mind. As medical professionals, prescribers and nurses are trained to do things. They aren't in the habit of just standing around and waiting, so don't expect them to do that. Instead, make sure they understand that in the case of presumed UTI (for example), they should push fluids, take vitals, and monitor the patient for any change in condition. What they *shouldn't* do is prescribe or give antibiotics unless they've determined that the patient meets the strict case definition for UTI. The same holds true for presumed pneumonia and presumed pressure wound infections.

DON'T AIM FOR A "ONE-AND-DONE"

After that first successful in-service, you could be forgiven for thinking the training was over. However, you'd be wrong. In fact, we scheduled a full series of in-service meetings. Look, introducing an antibiotic stewardship program like this is a paradigm shift for most people. They haven't done anything like this before, so a lot of the time, they don't even know what they don't know. Scheduling a series of in-service days for the entire staff gives everyone a chance to try out the new approach, find their sticking points, and get answers to the questions that inevitably come up.

To keep things manageable, I recommend breaking up the meetings to better serve each type of staff member. For example, at Devon Gables, we decided to work with NPs and the senior team in the morning, then the nurses and CNAs in the early afternoon, and all the ancillary staff in the late afternoon. Conducting the in-service meetings alongside the IP is also a good idea, because ultimately, the IP is the linchpin that holds the whole thing together. You want to make sure they understand what's going on, what issues the staff are facing, and how to solve them!

Don't get me wrong: you don't need to hold these in-service meetings in perpetuity. Conducting them once per week for four or six weeks is enough to get everyone started. Then, once you've collected your first quarter of data, you can hold a refresher session to share results and reacquaint everyone with the game plan moving forward. You can also use the in-service days to train everyone on the new policies you've put in place (decolonization, anyone?), so that you're ready the next time CMS comes knocking on your door.

Remember to check in with the IP once a month, too. Look at the data they've collected, review the trends with them, and decide whether you should stay on the same course or if a correction is in order. That's what I'll be doing at Devon Gables with Maricela over the next year, and it's what you should do at your facility when you start (or revive) your own antibiotic stewardship program.

KEEP THE DATA SEPARATE

I've said it before, and I'll say it again: Data is crucial to a strong antibiotic stewardship program. To be useful, though, your data needs to be accurate, and it needs to be clean. That's why I highly suggest you work with your IP to separate the data they collect for their infection prevention and control program from the data they collect for the stewardship program.

Prior to Devon Gables, I've always let the IPs use the same form for both types of data. Not anymore; the daily data they collect for the stewardship program should go on its own spreadsheet. Each month, we'll review the data and then present it to the Q/A committee at our monthly meeting. Following that meeting, Dr. Wadleigh and I will put together a transmittal memo that will go to all the prescribers highlighting the monthly results. As with everything else I've shared with you in this chapter, I suggest you do the same at your own facility. Of course, I don't advise getting too fixated on the monthly data—as I mentioned in chapter 4, trends are more important than individual month results—but the monthly transmittal memo reminds everyone that the game has new rules, and they better get with the program. Remember, antibiotics are deeply ingrained in our culture, so keeping your stewardship program at the forefront of everyone's minds will help ensure they maintain strict adherence to the case definitions (and, therefore, decrease the amount of "just in case" antibiotics that are prescribed).

GOING QUARTER BY QUARTER

Each time I meet with Devon Gables leadership and/or staff, I reiterate that the purpose of the stewardship program is to move the needle forward. We aren't going to solve the problem overnight, and it's not realistic to expect that we will. I recommend you make that clear to your staff and leadership, too. Then set goals for the upcoming quarter.

For example, the goal for our first quarter at Devon Gables is to identify one of the three or four practices that we want to interrupt. If the data ends up showing that only one case out of ten met the strict case definition for UTI, our goal will be to interrupt empiric prescribing (giving an antibiotic without first running a diagnostic test and waiting for the results) for UTIs. In other words, all the focus for that quarter will be on UTIs; we won't worry so much about presumed pneumonia or presumed pressure wound infections. Of course, that's not to say that we'll give nurses and prescribers carte blanche to ignore those case definitions, but our main focus will be on reducing empiric use of antibiotics for UTIs.

Once the data for the following quarter is in, we'll review it and see whether or not we made any progress in our target area. If so, we'll keep going until that issue is resolved, and then (and only then) move on to the next. If no progress was made, we'll dig into why and address the root causes of the issue, then review the following quarter's data to make sure our efforts have made a positive change before moving on. And of course, even after we've made progress in a given area, we'll continue to monitor the data quarterly to make sure there's no backsliding.

Obviously, the success of a program like this relies a great deal on accountability. It's important to remember, though, that you catch more flies with honey than vinegar. Trust me when I say that it's far more effective to invite people to climb aboard the stewardship train than to demand they do. If you try to coerce people to do things differently, especially pre-scribers, they usually end up digging their heels in, and then nothing gets done.

So how do you issue the invitation to play along? Partly by telling them the truth—the same truth I've shared with you throughout this book—and partly by showing them that you're on their side. One way to do this is to let them know there's a federal regulation now that requires you to set up an antibiotic stewardship program. Make sure the prescribers in particular know you fully believe they are committed to doing what's best for their patients, and make it clear that you are implementing this program to help them achieve that goal while still remaining in compliance with federal regulations. You can also share with them how much of a difference they will make in the long run when their patients finally experience freedom from the sickness that comes with overusing antibiotics. And you can show them the charts and numbers I've shared with you here, so they can see what's possible when they reduce their use of "just in case" antibiotics.

THE MIRACLE DRUG

During the in-service days, chances are you'll learn some things you might otherwise never have known about your staff. For example, Heather (the administrator at Devon Gables) told us at the first meeting that, many years ago, her mother cut her cheek on a rose bush in their garden. It was Kansas City in 1941, long before antibiotics were available to the general public. The cut got infected, and there was no penicillin available. Pretty soon, her mother was in the hospital, and the doctors were worried that she was going to die.

Hard to imagine now, right? But that was the reality in 1941: Even something as simple as a scratch from a rose bush

could kill you. Luckily, her doctor knew the people in a local laboratory. This particular lab was one of the first to manufacture penicillin in quantities sufficient to give to patients; her doctor persuaded the people in the lab to give him some penicillin, and it saved her life.

These days, antibiotics have become so deeply entrenched in our culture that we turn to them for every little thing. However, by implementing the antibiotic stewardship program I've described—just like I'm doing at Devon Gables— you can help turn the tide and keep antibiotics functioning as the miracle drugs they are so often hailed to be.

Now that you've seen how to launch a strong antibiotic stewardship program at a relatively large facility, let's turn our attention to a case study from another facility: Glencroft Center for Modern Aging. Unlike Devon Gables', Glencroft's program is well established, so—with the benefit of hindsight—we'll be able to see exactly what worked, what didn't, and why.

KEY TAKEAWAYS

- To maximize the effectiveness of your antibiotic stewardship program, prioritize a series of in-service training days for all of your staff (and the senior leadership team).

- Break down training sessions so staff members in similar roles engage in the training together.
- Remember that results don't happen overnight; focusing on a single goal each quarter will help keep the needle moving forward.

7

GLENCROFT

A T NEARLY 900 RESIDENTS, GLENCROFT CENTER
for Modern Aging is the largest continuing care retire-
ment community in Arizona. While it offers independent and assisted living, memory care, and long-term care, it
is also a single-location community. As such, it was the perfect place to "test drive" my antibiotic stewardship program
in a real-world situation, right from the first meeting to the
end of the first year. After all, the number of people we could
positively impact by focusing on Glencroft's population was a
chance to make forward progress in a significant way.

Remember earlier in the book when I told you about
Mary Matesan? If so, you may recall that she was one of the

original people who got me connected with Glencroft. Mary and I had known each other at Diagnostic Labs, so when she started working at Glencroft as the ADON, she called to ask if I would be willing to come to the facility and talk to the staff about antibiotics. Would I?!? Absolutely—I was thrilled to do it! And it was the perfect way to start the whole process. Education is the foundation of change, and Mary understood that on a deep level.

When I arrived to give my talk, the room was packed with people. Nurses, CNAs, and PAs filled the seats. The medical director, a woman named Dr. Marie Rink, was there, too. I opened the way I always do, telling the room the truth about antibiotics. Then after I had talked for about twenty minutes, we got into the Q&A portion of the show. Dr. Rink kicked things off with a practical question: "It's hard to get a clean-catch urine specimen from our residents. Any advice?"

It was a great question, and one that naturally led to a deeper issue: How, but also when, should facility personnel culture people for UTIs? I thought for a minute and then told her that a lot of the culture results I had seen were just colonization. That's how I thought about it back then: I wasn't yet thinking about the fact that asymptomatic colonization bacteria in the bladder with no symptoms is very common. I was just thinking about how to get the specimen properly so that the results would be accurate. Dr. Rink nodded, then said,

"You know, maybe we could do an in-and-out catheterization for everyone." Seeing that level of engagement was heartening, so I said, "You know, probably the best way to answer the question is to think about whether this is real bacteriuria in the bladder, or is it part of the colonization in the urethra on the way out?" My point was that it's the same as when you get a sputum specimen, too. You get a nice specimen but then drag it through the sewer that is the human mouth. As a result, when you put the specimen in a sputum cup, it's going to grow all sorts of things that don't truly reflect what's really going on with the patient.

The more we talked about it, the more we arrived at the conclusion that a urine dipstick urinalysis might be positive, but that doesn't necessarily mean infection. So eventually, I added another piece of advice—one that mirrors the UTI protocol I've shared with you already: Get a lot of fluid into the person you want to culture so there's no dark urine, then do the in-and-out catheterization Dr. Rink had suggested. Everyone in the room was nodding because they knew I was right, and the questions kept flowing.

It was a great start to the whole program, because everyone relaxed and realized that we were all there for the same thing: doing right by the residents. I wasn't there to shame them, or make them feel like they were doing things wrong. All I was doing was inviting them to approach things from a different perspective. Remember, when you change the way you look at things, the things you look at change; I was simply helping them look at things differently. Keep that in mind when you're introducing the idea of a new and improved stewardship program to your own facility. By inviting staff to row in a different direction than they have been so far, but to do so *with you*, you reduce any perception that you're a threat to them or their way of doing things. That will go a long way toward making sure everyone moves in lockstep.

Because that first talk was such a great success, the leadership at Glencroft were excited to move forward. Glencroft is huge, though, so we had to be savvy about how we approached implementation. We decided to start by focusing on their skilled nursing facility, which has about 180 beds. You may remember from previous chapters that during the fourth quarter of 2014, when we started, there were ninety-four urine C&S orders; sixty-five of them were positive. In the first quarter of 2015, the number of urine C&S orders had dropped to sixty-three, with forty-six of them positive. A year after we started, the number of urine C&S orders had reduced by almost *78 percent*, to twenty-one. Of the twenty-one orders, ten of those were positive (almost *85 percent* fewer positives than we'd had when we started).

Think about that for a moment: In only one year, we had reduced the number of orders by almost 78 percent, and the number of positives had gone down by nearly 85 percent. It gets better: The UTI antibiotic days of therapy had dropped from 285 to only 85. The number of *C. difficile* positives had gone from seven to zero. And the number of ESBL positives had gone from twenty-one to four.

I know I've shared this information with you previously, but I invite you to pause for a moment and reflect on these outcomes again. If Glencroft could see improvements like that in just one year, so can your facility. And believe me, when it does, the long-term impact for your residents will be staggering.

REDUCE UNNECESSARY ORDERS

So what was the secret to Glencroft's success? This is an especially compelling question, given that they've been in operation since the 1970s. Clearly, results like the ones we got in the first year of the program—more than 50 years after they were founded—didn't happen by accident. Once you understand how they achieved what they did, you can apply those same lessons to your own facility, strengthening your own program in the process.

One of the most important things Glencroft did was reduce the number of urine C&S orders. Far too often, when a urine C&S is ordered, the prescriber puts the patient on "just in case" antibiotics. It's a natural urge: The C&S was almost undoubtedly ordered in the first place because the resident had some confusion, or smelly urine, or "could just tell" they had a UTI. In other words, the presumption that the resident had a UTI was the basis for the order. And given what you know about how most prescribers treat antibiotics, what's the typical outcome when a prescriber assumes someone has a UTI? Ding ding ding! You guessed it—antibiotics.

Glencroft (and more specifically, Mary Matesan) put a stop to that. Because we were collecting data daily about C&S orders and days of therapy, Mary had the exact ammunition she needed to march up to anyone who issued an order and ask them, point-blank, why they had done so. Pretty soon, as I've mentioned before, people stopped doing cultures willy-nilly, because they knew they'd have to explain themselves to Mary. They started using the UTI protocol instead and only doing cultures when there was a solid reason for them. Furthermore, when cultures were performed, they waited to make sure the patient fit the strict case definition for UTI before putting them on antibiotics. That's why the days of therapy dropped from 268 to 85 in only a year.

You can do the same thing at your facility. Educate your IP about when it's appropriate for prescribers to order cultures and how nurses should talk to prescribers about presumed UTIs. Then empower them to hold prescribers and nurses accountable for their actions. Let them know that it's okay to ask prescribers and nurses point-blank, "Why did you order that culture? And why is that person on an antibiotic?" When you couple an IP like Mary Matesan with a deeply supportive medical director, the results are astounding. So create that dynamic: Support your IP in becoming another Mary Matesan, and before you know it, your antibiotic stewardship program will be flying high.

CHANGE THE CULTURE

More than half the residents at Glencroft are in independent living apartments. Your facility may be similar. If so, I'm sure you know that, unlike skilled nursing and assisted living, independent living is non-regulated. That can make things a bit harder when it comes to antibiotic stewardship, since you don't have the same regulations to fall back on that you do with other types of care. But all hope is not lost; you simply have to come at program implementation a different way.

At Glencroft and other facilities I've worked with, the answer to this quandary has been to change the culture. Remember how we started with the skilled nursing facility at Glencroft? After a year of really focusing on boosting their antibiotic stewardship program in the skilled nursing facility, we had changed the culture among the staff when it came to antibiotics.

Because of the work we did that first year, the staff were used to collecting data. They were used to defining their cases and reducing the number of cultures ordered. And they could see, plain as the noses on their faces, that the vast majority of patients in the skilled nursing facility had been given antibiotics for infections they simply did not have. Once they understood that—and saw how much antibiotic resistance started to unwind when "just in case" antibiotics were reduced—it carried over into how they dealt with residents in the rest of the community, including the independent living folks.

To make it really effective, bolster a change in culture with your data. Once people can see with their own two eyes that positive results show up when the number of cultures goes down, they can understand, on a visceral level, how what they're doing is working. And when you send out updates and reports every month with the latest data, that momentum is sustained. People want to continue making a positive difference, and pretty soon, they've stopped pulling cultures and prescribing antibiotics for residents who don't fulfill defined criteria for UTI.

The data can also work to show people what not to do. To show you what I mean, let's zoom in from the 30,000-foot view and look at a single patient's antibiotic journey from 2013 through 2015:

Antibiotic Journey (2013–2015)

Date of Service	Organism/ Colony Count	Clinical	Rx	Comment
2/26/2013	*Providencia stuartii:* 25,000 cfu/ml	Screening UA negative		Gentamicin peak/trough 2/16 and 2/18/2013
8/17/2013	*E. coli:* 50,000 cfu/ml			
12/9/2013	*E. coli:* >100,000 cfu/ml			
12/26/2013	*E. coli:* >100,000 cfu/ml			
5/14/2014	*E. coli:* >100,000 cfu/ml		Nitrofurantoin x 10 days	Gentamicin peak/trough 5/29
8/8/2014	*E. coli:* >100,000 cfu/ml	Patient lethargic; started Abx; C&S ordered	Nitrofurantoin x 10 days	
9/16/2014	*E. coli:* 50,000 cfu/ml	"urine foul"	Nitrofurantoin x 10 days	
10/1/2014	*E. coli:* 50,000 cfu/ml *P. aeruginosa:* 50,000 cfu/ml		Gentamicin	Gentamicin peak/trough 10/14/2014
10/26/2014	*MR S. Aureus:* 50,000 cfu/ml *Enterococcus:* 50,000 cfu/ml			"s/p gent for UTI"
10/26/2014	*Pr. Mirabilis:* 50,000 cfu/ml *Gm + cocci:* <10,000 cfu/ml			
3/17/2015	*Pr. Mirabilis:* >100,000 cfu/ml *Gm + cocci:* <10,000 cfu/ml			*C. difficile,* stool C&S, O&P negative

Looking at the first line, you can see that the *Providencia stuartii* colony count is insignificant. The UA screening was also negative. Clearly, this person didn't have a UTI; they had asymptomatic bacteriuria. But clearly, the prescriber decided to use antibiotics "just in case" by treating this patient intravenously with gentamicin. That's a pretty powerful antibiotic, especially when it's used to treat an infection that isn't actually there!

Not even a year later, the patient was cultured and found to have *E. coli* >100,000 cfu/ml. Now, I know what you're thinking: the *E. coli* was over 100,000. It's got to be treated!

Not so fast. Remember, the *only* time antibiotics should be prescribed for UTI is when the patient meets the strict case definition...and that requires more than *E. coli* over 100,000 cfu/ml. If you see something like this in your own facility, get your IP to investigate. That's the best way to prevent what happened to this patient: Over the next five months, the patient was treated for UTIs they didn't have. And they got six cultures for UTI in 2014 alone! It was a classic case of empirical antibiotic therapy—the very thing that a good antibiotic stewardship program seeks to rule out. However, the story this data shows is far from unique: The average nursing home resident gets five or six cultures per year, with some people getting twice that number.

Granted, this patient wasn't at Glencroft, but they are representative of how Glencroft approached cultures and antibiotic prescribing before I came onto the scene in 2014. Chances are, this kind of scenario is representative of how things play out for your residents, too. That's why it's so important to utilize data to change the culture around antibiotic stewardship in your facility. By making sure people think about why they're doing a culture before they do it, you can eliminate a lot of unnecessary prescribing. And by making it instinctive for people to pump the brakes before they start tossing antibiotics around like candy, you can help reduce any instances of "just in case" antibiotics for the cultures that are performed—not just for skilled nursing residents, but for people in every part of your facility (even the non-regulated sections).

So far, we've looked at what's entailed in launching an antibiotic stewardship program at a smaller facility and what helped make the stewardship program at a large facility a rousing success. Now, let's consider what it might look like to implement a stewardship program in a multifacility network. This is especially important because there are certain pitfalls that come along with networks that you won't run into elsewhere. Forewarned is forearmed, as they say, so let's arm you with the information you need to make a multifacility network program a success. Here we go!

KEY TAKEAWAYS

- Invite your staff to think of the antibiotic stewardship program as a way to come together to better serve the residents. Making this a collaborative process will help reduce dissension and keep everyone moving forward together.
- Reducing the number of urine C&S orders is crucial to ensuring your antibiotic stewardship program succeeds.
- Empower your IP to question why cultures were taken and antibiotics were prescribed.
- Weaving antibiotic stewardship into your facility's culture is key to the program's long-term and continued success.

8

COVENANT HEALTH NETWORK

A FEW YEARS AFTER I HELPED GLENCROFT TAKE their antibiotic stewardship program to the level they aspired to, I was approached by Covenant Health Network (Covenant). They had heard about what I had helped Glencroft accomplish, and they wanted me to help them achieve something similar. There was only one problem: they were a multifacility network, which was a completely different beast from Glencroft (even as large as it was). Each facility within Covenant's network was connected administratively, but they each had their own teams, their own staff, and their own leadership. It was daunting, but it was also a chance to implement better antibiotic stewardship from the ground up for a large number of facilities at once, so I agreed.

Before we dive into what worked, what didn't, and why, let me give you a little more context about the project. With eleven facilities in Arizona (all of which are local to Phoenix, where I live), thirteen in Colorado, eleven in Mississippi, thirty-five in Pennsylvania, and one in New Mexico, we were dealing with a *big* network of facilities that offered everything from skilled nursing to memory care, assisted living, and independent living. To make things a bit more manageable, we decided to start with the eleven Arizona facilities. I recommend, if you are involved with a multifacility network, that you do the same. Breaking things into bite-sized chunks gives you a chance to iron out the kinks before you roll out network-wide, increasing your chances of success and ensuring your program runs as smoothly as possible.

LOOK AT THE DATA

Every program has to start somewhere, so initially, I went out to Covenant's headquarters in Phoenix and gave a talk at their regular health care meeting. The senior leadership for each of their facilities were in the room, and I talked to them all about the importance of antibiotic stewardship. Like I had done a hundred times before, I shared the truth about antibiotics with them and talked to them about how we are dangerously close to going over the post-antibiotic cliff. Then I told them that, because they were such a large network, there was a good chance they could be instrumental in helping us pull back from the abyss. They were sold: step one—getting leadership buy-in and alignment—was complete.

We started the antibiotic stewardship program in 2016. A year later, we had our results. While not quite as impressive as Glencroft's, we had made good headway. More importantly, we had learned some key lessons about what to do *and* what not to do to make multifacility stewardship programs successful. I'll share those lessons with you here, but first, let's look at the data (on the following page).

As you can see, when we started in 2016, the number of urine C&S orders was a whopping eighty-three. That number dropped drastically the next quarter, to fifty-five. By the end of one year, it had reduced to thirty-six. That was an almost 57 percent decrease! Not bad, especially given the challenges we faced. Even more heartening: by the time we finished the first year, the number of positive cultures almost exactly matched the number of cultures performed. In other words, cultures weren't being performed for no good reason. In almost every instance, they were valid. Compare that to the first quarter of 2017, when fifty-five cultures were performed and only twenty-eight were positive. In light of numbers like that, it was clear that we had made good progress in one short year, which spoke to the quality of the program we had put into place.

Antibiotic Stewardship Metrics

Name of Network: Covenant Health Network
Reporting Period: Calendar Year 2017

Metric	4Q 2016	1Q 2017	2Q 2017	3Q 2017	4Q 2017
Urine C&S orders	83	55	47	41	36
Urine C&S positive		28	33	32	34
Antibiotic Rx		31	40	35	30
Rx with low colony count or multiple organisms		7	21	15	16
Meeting standardized clinical criteria		24	19	20	12
Antibiotic Rx empiric (before C&S result)		5	4	12	3
Days of Antibiotic Therapy (DOT)	357	312	273	236	171
Days of Inappropriate Therapy (IDOT)		88	98	55	77
C. difficile orders		7	3	1	2
C. difficile positive		2	0	1	1
ESBL + urine isolates		5	2	5	2

Some other highlights revealed by the data: the number of days of antibiotic therapy started out at 357. By the fourth quarter of 2017, it had dropped over 50 percent, to 171. The number of days of inappropriate therapy had dropped from eighty-eight to fifty-five, which was a decrease of 37.5 percent. The number of *C. difficile* cases had gone from two to just one, and the number of ESBL positives had dropped from five to two.

At the end of the year, a memo went out detailing the results of the first year of our antibiotic stewardship program. Sent by Matt Luger, CEO of Covenant, the memo stated that "initial indications from the antibiotic stewardship program show promising outcomes, as facilities, nurses, and medical practitioners are educated on how to correctly identify and treat (or not treat) positive urine cultures. [...] Overall reduction in the use of antibiotics has been shown to reduce the incidence of *C. difficile* in the aging population." Clearly, they were happy, and for the most part, so was I.

WHAT WORKED...

My experience at Covenant affirmed that education is one of the most important components of a strong antibiotic stewardship program. With the help of key Covenant staff, including Trish Manchester, RN (Covenant's director of quality initiatives), I conducted approximately twenty training sessions for the program participants. I also conducted additional outreach for each facility's attending physicians and medical directors—remember, prescriber buy-in is key!

However, given the sheer number of facilities we were working with, we knew we needed to do more than just conduct training sessions. So Trish created a "Best Practices Antibiotic Stewardship" manual. This manual reflected the most current antibiotic stewardship research, literature, and policies, and was supplied to all facilities both in hard copy and on a jump drive. Offering the manual in both formats made it easier for facilities to utilize and share the information provided in the manual, which increased staff members' adherence to and understanding of the program.

Because we were working with a large number of facilities spread across the entire state of Arizona, we had to hold the training sessions remotely. This was in prehistoric times before Zoom and similar programs were widely utilized, so we had to hold the sessions via an internal corporate video call system. It was clunky, but it was the only way to disseminate information in the way it needed to be shared. It worked, up to a point, but it also had some shortcomings... ones you'll need to overcome if you run a multifacility network. Let me explain.

AND WHAT DIDN'T

One of the biggest challenges we faced with the technology available at the time was how hard it was for people to truly participate. Nowadays, with Zoom, everyone in a facility can simply take their phone out or log onto a computer and join the call. Not back then. Because the video call system was connected to a monitor and required a line to dial in, people had to make their way to a specific conference room at the time the meeting was being held. Then they had to pack into said conference room like sardines. It was uncomfortable, to say the least, and the result was that, at any given training, a significant number of staff simply didn't show up.

Look, if you want your stewardship program to work (or any program, for that matter), *you have to make it easy for people to do the right thing and hard for them to do the wrong thing.* At Covenant, there was simply too much leeway for people to skip the calls. I'm sure I don't have to tell you that everyone at a facility is busy, so if they don't have to be at a training session, or if attending it is hard, then more often than not, they'll skip it.

The other issue is that, often, the staff who were missing from the trainings were key to the success of the antibiotic stewardship program. To be more specific, the IPs and the UA nurses regularly missed calls. It's hard to keep an antibiotic stewardship program running if key people only show up every third or fourth meeting! Think about it: if someone only comes sporadically, when they *do* show up, you're busy answering questions that you already answered previously, which means your time isn't used effectively. It's a huge problem and will impact your program dramatically.

Don't get me wrong: I'm not disparaging Covenant's staff. They were incredibly busy and hard-working people. However, that doesn't change the fact that for an antibiotic stewardship program to work, you need people to commit their time and resources to it. So how do you do that?

The solution is multifold. First and foremost, if you're training people at a variety of locations, utilize a program like Zoom to make it easy for them to attend, no matter where they are or what they're doing. Second, make it mandatory for them to be there. Third, set a rhythm for your training sessions, just like I described in the chapter at Devon Gables, and stick to it.

Another issue we ran into was getting equal buy-in across facilities. Some of the CEOs were very much on board. Others were less so. So take the time to build relationships with all the CEOs in your network. If a facility isn't performing to the same standards as others, the data will reflect that. In those instances, focus on the facility that's struggling. Work directly with its leadership to make sure they understand what's at stake, what the goals are, and why they should care. Then make sure their staff understands the same things. This may require additional education sessions, more focused collaboration with their IP, or something else. Every situation is unique, but if you remember to make antibiotic stewardship an invitation and a collaboration, you'll be able to get the job done. And once you build that initial momentum, you're halfway there.

Once a facility's leadership team is on board, you'll be able to overcome the final obstacle we faced at Covenant. In a nutshell, many of the network's facilities seemed to view participation in the stewardship program as something that was voluntary. To be really effective, the program needs to be a mandate, like it is at Devon Gables. The foundation for making the mandate clear is the signed announcement letter, so make sure the staff and prescribers at every facility in your network receive a letter signed by their senior leadership team. This will run the new protocol up the flagpole, so to speak, and serve as a clear indication that things are going to change—and they need to act accordingly.

ADDRESS THE BIG THREE

Finally, keep the program's focus on the big three: presumed UTI, presumed pneumonia, and presumed pressure wound infections. If you do that, you give people something concrete to really sink their teeth into without overwhelming them. It's no exaggeration to say that, if you focus on the big three, you'll be operating above the 99th percentile when it comes to antibiotic stewardship. And as you've seen over and over, when you focus on these three culprits, the world will change. The degree of multiple resistance will go down at every facility in your network, just as it did at Covenant.

Now that we've looked at several case studies, you have a better sense of what to do and what not to do when you're starting (or reviving) your own antibiotic stewardship program. So let's finish out the discussion by turning our attention to a few more pitfalls that you might encounter on your journey, and what to do about them.

KEY TAKEAWAYS

- Education is one of the most important components of a multifacility antibiotic stewardship program.
- Creating a "best practices" manual will help ensure everyone in the network has the information they need to support the stewardship program.
- Utilize technology like Zoom to make your training sessions easily accessible.
- Make it mandatory for staff, especially key personnel like IPs, to attend every single training session.
- Spend the time necessary to get each individual facility's leadership on board and ensure their alignment with the program.

- When you're implementing and running your program, keep your focus on the big three: presumed UTI, presumed pneumonia, and presumed pressure wound infections.

9

AVOIDING THE
PITFALLS

A S YOU IMPLEMENT YOUR ANTIBIOTIC STEWARD-
ship, there's one question I want you to ask yourself
regularly: Is what we're doing working? If the answer
is no, then another question needs to be asked: What do you
need to change to move the needle in the right direction?

There are all kinds of reasons why your antibiotic stewardship program might not be getting the results you want.
Remember, when it's working, the first thing that happens
is the number of urine cultures decreases. Pretty soon, the
number of days of antibiotic therapy starts going down. And
then if you've been tracking multidrug resistance (and you

should be), you'll notice that will start to unwind, because your stewardship program is interrupting the stimulus fueling it—namely, the rampant overuse of antibiotics. All of these results should be noticeable within the first quarter, if not the first month. If they aren't, there's a problem.

Before we dive into some of the most common pitfalls and what to do about them, I think it's important to discuss why stewardship programs work so quickly. This is also helpful information to share with your staff during one of your education sessions, so they understand why it's reasonable to expect to see results so quickly. Essentially, the organisms we're talking about divide at an incredibly rapid rate. Some of them move to a new generation every twenty minutes. So when you change any of the stimuli affecting these organisms—for example, you stop giving antibiotics—the resulting change shows up quickly. Granted, this is a simplified way of explaining things, but it drives home the point that any changes you make start to impact future generations of organisms almost immediately. So if you don't see changes, something is wrong with your program.

BEWARE THE GUNSLINGERS

One of the biggest reasons antibiotic stewardship programs fail is because staff members and prescribers don't strictly adhere to case definitions when prescribing and giving antibiotics. So that's the first thing to check anytime your data doesn't show progress. Have your infection preventionist talk to the nurses. The goal of those discussions? To find out if one (or more) prescribers is shooting from the hip when it comes to antibiotics. The nurses will know, and they'll probably tell the IP about a prescriber who habitually puts a patient on ceftriaxone or some other intravenous antibiotic the minute a nurse reports that the patient is confused or has what the nurse deems to be "foul urine."

When you hear about a prescriber like this, chances are they didn't fully understand or believe what the announcement letter said. So have the medical director talk to them. Make sure the prescriber understands they *must* adhere to a strict case definition before prescribing antibiotics for any of the big three. Fall back on federal regulations if you need to. As I've previously mentioned, it's always best to make it an invitation, but at the end of the day, be very clear: The old guard has left the building, there's a new sheriff in town, and they need to act accordingly.

WATCH FOR BACKSLIDES

The longer I've been at this, the more I've come to realize that, many times, problems don't emerge right away. In fact, for the first few quarters, it's far more common to see amazing results. Then, slowly, the results get less and less impressive, until suddenly, a year or eighteen months in, you're back where you started. Why? Because at the start of something, everyone is gung-ho about it. They're excited, they're aligned, and as a result, they nail it. But then, the excitement wears off, the focus shifts elsewhere, and they fall back into their old habits.

I think about antibiotic stewardship like a campfire: if you don't keep feeding it, it will go out. And it takes a lot more effort to relight a fire that's died than to keep it going in the first place.

So don't let your fire die. Use your monthly meetings and transmittal memos to keep antibiotic stewardship at the front of everyone's mind. Anytime a new prescriber comes onboard, give them an orientation that talks about antibiotic stewardship, why it's so important, and what's expected of them. You can give them a "best practices" manual like the one Covenant Health Network created to answer their questions and drive home how important it is for them to adhere to the program. And you can send out a report letter every year outlining what happened over the past twelve months. In the letter, congratulate everyone for the accomplishments they made, then share your plan for the coming year. Have your senior leadership team sign the annual report letter, just as they did the announcement letter, and publish it widely in your facility.

We've talked about this previously, but the importance of taking actions like these simply cannot be overstated. Keep talking about your program, keep managing your program, and keep making antibiotic stewardship a foundational part of your culture. If you do, then chances are high your program will maintain momentum far into the future.

LABORATORIES

While it's likely you have a specific laboratory you've been working with for a long time, getting the right laboratory on board is key to ensuring your stewardship program is a success. That's why it's worth discussing some criteria I look for when determining whether or not a lab is doing a good job. First of all, make sure your laboratory runs on the principles of clinically relevant microbiology. If they don't, then I can guarantee you they will contribute to your overuse of antibiotics.

One of the best ways to do this is to talk to the laboratory director. Can they answer clinical questions? Do they know the truth about antibiotics and resistance? What is their response when you discuss stewardship with them? Are they tied to symptom-focused case definitions?

Along with asking questions like these, you should also discuss the minimal inhibitory concentration (MIC) for an antibiotic with your laboratory. Some lab reports include the role of MICs next to the antibiotics, which can lead to erroneous decision-making by the clinician. They think the MIC numbers mean the correct antibiotic is the one with the lowest MIC, which is completely false. Using the MIC to choose the antibiotic is incorrect, so take the time to discuss MICs with the lab director. Then make sure your prescribers understand that, no matter what the lab reports show, they should ignore MICs for urine and wound cultures. In fact, they should ignore MICs for *anything* that isn't normally sterile. Including a policy around minimal criteria for antibiotic therapy is helpful to give nurses and prescribers something to reference. To ensure the widest dissemination, the medical director can include the MIC policy in their monthly report, along with a reminder to all prescribers about what the minimal criteria is and the importance of making sure a patient matches the case definition before prescribing an antibiotic.

One more thing to check for when you're thinking about the quality of your lab: turnaround time. For urine cultures, turnaround time shouldn't be longer than forty-eight hours; a few hours is better (remember, these organisms divide really quickly). X-rays should be turned around within a day. And of course, make sure they couple that fast turnaround time with accurate (i.e., clinically relevant) results.

ARM YOUR STAFF WITH KNOWLEDGE

Remember at the beginning of the book when we talked about how lots of people insist their loved one can *just tell* when they have a UTI? Well, that leads us to another common pitfall: giving in to family or resident pressure for antibiotics against the nurse's or prescriber's better judgment. To address this particular pitfall, educate your residents and their families. Pass out the short article "Are You Sure Your Loved One Has A UTI?" (included in chapter 1) to all your residents and their families, and include it in the welcome package for new residents. You can also ask your residents and their family members to take the pledge to become antibiotic guardians (also included in chapter 1). Taking steps like these will bolster your program by making everyone—not just the staff or the prescribers, but residents and families, too—a participant.

When you arm your staff with knowledge and empower them to stand firm in antibiotic stewardship, you help to head off another potential pitfall: maintaining stewardship in the event of a COVID or other infectious disease outbreak. Look, if your facility is going through an outbreak, it's hard to keep the momentum going for antibiotic stewardship. However, if your staff members are cross-trained to handle different parts of the program, there's a much higher likelihood appropriate data will still get collected and key metrics will still get

BECOMING GOOD STEWARDS OF ANTIBIOTICS

measured and reported. So identify who needs to be trained in what, build in redundancies, and spell everything out in your antibiotic stewardship program policy.

These are some of the most common pitfalls that frequently occur; odds are you'll encounter others in your antibiotic stewardship journey. So that's why my final piece of advice to you is to remember the PDCA cycle (PDCA stands for plan, do, check, act). Set up your plan, execute it, check the results, and then act to revise it as necessary. If you stay alert and open-minded, you'll continuously find ways to improve upon what you're doing. When I first started helping people implement antibiotic stewardship programs, for example, I didn't instruct them to send out an announcement letter that had been signed by the entire senior leadership team. It was only signed by the medical director. We noticed we were having trouble getting buy-in, so we decided to add more signatories, and the results were impressive. Now, getting the letter signed by the medical director, the administrator, the DON, and the IP is a core element of each antibiotic stewardship program I consult on, and I hope it will be a core element of yours.

Ultimately, your antibiotic stewardship will be exactly as good as you make it. When you're committed to it, and you get buy-in from leadership and staff for it, you have every-thing you need to positively impact antibiotic overuse in your facility.

Congratulations! You're almost ready to start (or revive) your own program. Before I send you off to do that, though, I want to share a few more thoughts with you about antibiotic stewardship—specifically, antibiotic stewardship in your facility. Let's do it!

KEY TAKEAWAYS

- As you implement your antibiotic stewardship program, continually ask yourself if what you're doing is working.
- If the answer is no, think about what you need to change to move the needle forward.
- Don't get complacent: stay alert for backsliding as your program matures.
- Arming your staff with knowledge and building in redundancies are good ways to avoid pitfalls and ensure your program's success.

Conclusion

THE CALL
TO ACTION

Over the course of the book, you've learned why antibiotic stewardship is so important. You've gained insight into what goes into a strong antibiotic stewardship program, and you've seen how various long-term care facilities have started or revived their own programs. You've also gotten a glimpse of some of the challenges that commonly plague antibiotic stewardship programs and gained practical knowledge about how to avoid these pitfalls.

Now it's time to put everything you've learned into practice. But before you do, I want to ask you a question: If there were no laws and regulations, and world-class quality was your goal, how much of what I've shared would you elect *not* to do?

On the surface, it might seem like a strange question, but humor me. If you didn't have to do antibiotic stewardship, how much of the advice in this book would you ignore? Because I'll tell you right now: If you want your program to succeed, simply maintaining compliance with regulations is the bottom of what's acceptable; it's the floor.

The ceiling, though? That doesn't have a limit. So continually move toward the apex, always, because every step you take on the road to better stewardship helps your residents get better care. That, in turn, ensures they'll stay healthier, both now and well into the future.

I'M ISSUING A CALL TO ACTION

This entire book has been a call to action. It's an invitation to you to encourage your residents and their loved ones—and, through them, your community at large—to become antibiotic guardians. Asking your residents and their families to sign the antibiotic pledge I shared in the first chapter is an honorable and effective way to disrupt conventional ways of thinking about antibiotics and introduce something new. Something better.

The book is a call to action for your facility's health care professionals, too. Their invitation is to become good stewards of antibiotics: to take intentional steps to move the needle toward more responsible antibiotic use. Specifically, it's an appeal for prescribers, nurses, and CNAs—as well as senior leadership—to stop using antibiotics indiscriminately and instead to only utilize them if someone meets the strict case definition for an infection. And it's a plea that health care professionals in long-term care facilities will stop giving in to patient pressure to use an antibiotic when the prescriber or nurse knows it won't do any good.

It's also an invitation to infection preventionists, administrators, and medical directors to start honing in on the right data: to examine *what* was being treated every time an antibiotic was prescribed, whether it was an *actual* infection, *how many days* someone was given antibiotic therapy, what *percentage of diagnoses* were true infections, and *how many people* received antibiotics for infections they didn't have. And it's a call for them to share that data with prescribers and other staff members, every single quarter, to help ensure the program's forward momentum is maintained.

Most of all, this book is an invitation for each and every one of us to alter our mindsets. To change the way we look at things so that the things we look at change. To recognize that we are teetering dangerously close to the post-antibiotic era and to do everything we can to prevent that from becoming our reality.

TOGETHER, WE CAN DO IT

I'm not saying that any of this will be easy. Quite the oppo-
site, in fact: There are barriers to achieving all of these
goals. Take prescribers, for example. I'm a doctor, so I can
tell you from personal experience that us physicians don't
take kindly to being coerced into doing things differently.
To paraphrase that famous song, the mindset amongst most
prescribers is, "It's my patient, and I'll do what I want to."
It's almost an unwritten law: Never interfere with another
doctor's orders, no matter how inappropriate or asinine
they may be. To a certain extent, I understand that mindset, but I also know it's a double-edged sword. If what a
prescriber wants to do is empirically prescribe antibiotics,
they're causing harm.

To create change, share the truth of antibiotics with them.
Make them understand that there are regulations in place
now to stop those sorts of practices. Even more than that,
help them see that they have a moral obligation *not* to do
harm. Ask them to join the movement to reduce antibiotic
overuse, even if it seems annoying or hard or unnecessary
to them. Most of all, make it easy for them to do the right
thing. If you can do all of this—and at the same time, make
doing the wrong thing akin to pushing a boulder uphill—then
before you know it, positive changes will occur.

The same is true for residents and their families. Remember the "elevator ambush" I described in chapter 1? It's a real thing, as I'm sure you know. The challenge is to eliminate the mindset that sparks those ambushes and replace it with an antibiotic guardian mindset. It requires patience, education, and compassion, but it can be done. I know, because I've seen it happen in every facility where I've consulted.

The stark reality is that long-term care facilities are awash in antibiotics. Residents average three or four courses of antibiotics per year. And with every round of unnecessary antibiotics, their sensitivity goes down and their resistance goes up. No single person or profession is to blame for this—every single one of us is guilty of overusing antibiotics, especially for self-limiting or viral infections like the flu or bronchitis. However, together, with the right mindset and the right focus, we can create change.

KEEP THE TRUTH IN MIND

Ultimately, this book is an invitation to keep the truth of antibiotics in mind. Remember, the primary problem with infectious disease today is people receiving antibiotics for infections they don't have. Don't be fooled when you hear "experts" saying more research is needed to find the root cause of antibiotic resistance. Don't fall for the idea that we don't know how to fix antibiotic resistance, either. Neither of those things are true.

With the right mindset, a sense of urgency, a deep commitment to the truth, and unwavering perseverance, we can avoid the post-antibiotic catastrophe lurking just around the bend. And we must—for all of us.

ACKNOWLEDGMENTS

Over the course of my career, I've been fortunate enough to work with some amazing people and institutions. Each of them, in their own way, informed my understanding of and approach to antibiotic stewardship. While I can't name them all here, I do want to take a moment to acknowledge those that played the biggest role in bringing the antibiotic stewardship program I've described in this book to life.

Thank you to Mary Matesan for wholeheartedly championing antibiotic stewardship—and making sure your staff did, too.

Thank you to my "inside person," Trish Manchester. You carried the ball when I couldn't be there, and in doing so, made sure the stewardship program kept going.

Thank you to Susan Brenner. You helped me figure out how to get the top people in the region on board. Because of you, we were able to overcome a lot of obstacles facing anti-biotic stewardship.

Thank you to Doug Maxwell. You helped me identify the structure of the implementation sequence. For that (and so many other things), I will always be grateful.

Thank you to Da Armenta, Debbie Friebus, and Maricela Nuñez. You are all some of the best infection preventionists I've ever had the honor to work with. Your commitment to antibiotic stewardship is second to none.

Thank you to Dr. Kate Ellingson for your excitement about and understanding of antibiotic stewardship. The work you are doing is changing lives.

Thank you to Dolly Greene. In every way, you truly are "Super Nurse."

Thank you to Diagnostic Laboratories & Radiology for being the place where it all started.

And finally, thank you to the facilities who let us test and perfect the antibiotic stewardship program described in this book: Glencroft Center for Modern Aging, Covenant Health Network, Devon Gables Rehabilitation Center, and University of Arizona – Mel & Enid Zuckerman College of Public Health.

ABOUT THE AUTHOR

Doctor Patterson, a.k.a. "Dr. Pete," is a third-generation physician who has been in practice for nearly 50 years. He began his career at Mile 49 of the Alaska Highway in 1969. After general practice, he trained in pathology and laboratory medicine, spending much of his career as a hospital pathologist, working behind the microscope and directing clinical laboratories. He began working in post-acute facilities in 2012 as lab director of a mobile diagnostics company, serving nursing homes and long-term care facilities.

Dr. Pete received his MD from the University of Alberta. In the past, he worked for a Fortune 500 health care manufacturing company, where he was trained in the principles and methods of Lean continuous quality improvement. He brings the perspectives of a practicing physician-manager to his current work as an author and consultant to long-term care facilities and networks.

Over the years, Dr. Pete has acquired an extensive background in medical quality improvement, clinical microbiology, and infection prevention/antibiotic stewardship. He has worked with many post-acute and long-term care facilities developing a results-oriented antibiotic stewardship protocol that has had a major positive impact on prescribing practices in skilled nursing facilities. In 2016, the protocol won a best-practice award from the California chapter of AMDA: the Society for Post-acute and Long-term Care Medicine.

He is a frequently invited speaker at conferences and provider network continuing education meetings. His on-the-ground practice experience and creative insights facilitate the transition in antibiotic prescribing mindset now underway in health care.

Dr. Pete currently lives in Phoenix, Arizona, with his wife, Margaret.